Vigorous Reforms

Vigorous Reforms
Women Writers and the Politics of Health in the Nineteenth-Century United States

Jess Libow

The University of North Carolina Press   CHAPEL HILL

© 2025 Jess Libow
All rights reserved
Set in Merope Basic by Westchester Publishing Services
Manufactured in the United States of America

Complete Cataloging-in-Publication Data for this title is available from the Library of Congress at https://lccn.loc.gov/2025013868.
ISBN 978-1-4696-8902-9 (cloth: alk. paper)
ISBN 978-1-4696-8903-6 (pbk.: alk. paper)
ISBN 978-1-4696-8310-2 (epub)
ISBN 978-1-4696-8904-3 (pdf)

Cover art: Photograph of a woman exercising. American Institute of Physical Culture (Medical Trade Ephemera). Courtesy of the Historical Medical Library of the College of Physicians of Philadelphia.

This book will be made open access within three years of publication thanks to Path to Open, a program developed in partnership between JSTOR, the American Council of Learned Societies (ACLS), the University of Michigan Press, and the University of North Carolina Press to bring about equitable access and impact for the entire scholarly community, including authors, researchers, libraries, and university presses around the world. Learn more at https://about.jstor.org/path-to-open/.

For product safety concerns under the European Union's General Product Safety Regulation (EU GPSR), please contact "mailto:gpsr@mare-nostrum.co.uk"gpsr@mare-nostrum.co.uk or write to the University of North Carolina Press and Mare Nostrum Group B.V., Mauritskade 21D, 1091 GC Amsterdam, The Netherlands.

Vigorous Reforms tells, among other things, a story about education. It is fitting, then, that teaching and learning from my students has sustained me throughout the writing process. This book is dedicated to them. Thank you for bringing your whole selves to the classroom and for your willingness to learn from one another.

Contents

List of Illustrations ix
Acknowledgments xi

Introduction 1

CHAPTER ONE
The Future of White Womanhood in Young America 14

CHAPTER TWO
Household Health in the Domestic's Novel 37

CHAPTER THREE
Harriet Jacobs and the Abolitionist "Science of Good Management" 58

CHAPTER FOUR
Pedagogies of Disability at the Carlisle Indian Industrial School 80

CHAPTER FIVE
"Education for Citizenship" and the Immigrant Body 100

Epilogue
From Physical Education to Wellness 127

Notes 137
Bibliography 169
Index 189

Illustrations

Students and teachers gathered outside the Jacobs School 76

Girls' gymnastics class at the Carlisle Indian Industrial School 84

Girls laundering at the Carlisle Indian Industrial School 88

Acknowledgments

As I often discuss with my students, writing is a long and collaborative process, and this book is no exception. These acknowledgments name only a few of the many people whose support made this project possible.

I could not have asked for a better editor than Lucas Church at the University of North Carolina Press. His enthusiasm about this project reinvigorated my own, and I am beyond grateful for his attunement to the challenges of writing and publishing a book as a contingent faculty member. I am also grateful to the two anonymous readers—who I was delighted to learn were Sari Edelstein and Sara Crosby—for believing that this manuscript could be a book and for the insights that helped it become one. Thank you as well to Thomas Bedenbaugh, Erin Granville, Lindsay Star, Alyssa Brown, and everyone else I've had the pleasure of working with at UNC Press.

I received support for this project from the Library Company of Philadelphia; the Historical Society of Pennsylvania; the College of Physicians of Philadelphia; the American Antiquarian Society; and the Consortium for History of Science, Technology, and Medicine. I am indebted to the staff at these institutions for their expertise and guidance—especially Connie King at the Library Company, who first showed me the ropes of archival research. I am grateful, too, to the editors and anonymous reviewers at *Legacy: A Journal of American Women Writers* and *J19: The Journal of Nineteenth-Century Americanists*, whose careful and generative comments helped shape chapters 1 and 3, respectively. I also want to thank Kostis Kourelis for inviting me to share part of this work at Franklin & Marshall College's 2024 symposium on *The Art of Unhealth*.

This book was shaped under the guidance of my mentors at Emory University. Since becoming my adviser without my even having to ask, Ben Reiss has remained firmly in my corner at every turn, pushing me to sharpen my arguments and to clarify the stakes of this project. At Emory, I also had the opportunity to work with one of my earliest influences, Rosemarie Garland-Thomson, whose support has been invaluable. Sander Gilman provided incisive feedback, persistently pushing me to see the bigger picture. Lauren Klein arrived on campus just when I needed her, and this book would not have been possible without her advice and her example. Both the

Disability Studies Initiative and the Writing Program provided intellectual community, and I am grateful for Paul Kelleher's and Dave Fisher's kindness and collegiality. Though we overlapped at Emory only briefly, Sari Altschuler has generously remained a mentor, and I have benefited immensely from her guidance.

Friends I met at Emory have also buoyed me along the way, and I had the privilege of developing the ideas in this book while learning alongside colleagues, including—but certainly not limited to—my cohort of Julian Currents, Joe Fritsch, Connor Larsen, Sophia Leonard Falvey, Will Parshley, Kayla Shipp, and William Tolbert. Sophia and Connor each deserve a special shout-out for walking and talking through the writing process with me. Marlo Starr, too, has been a true bud. Research trips to Massachusetts were enhanced by time spent with both Justin Shaw and Tesla Cariani. Thank you, Rachel Kolb, for so many thoughtful conversations and for your endless patience with my clumsy signing. I am also grateful for Jareka Dellenbaugh-Dempsey's friendship, which has bolstered me at crucial moments. It would be impossible to adequately thank Lindsey Grubbs, who reads drafts of nearly everything I write (including these acknowledgments) and whose friendship sustained me in so many ways as I was writing this book.

I am also indebted to colleagues at Haverford College. It has been a sincere pleasure to work alongside the brilliant scholars and teachers in the Haverford Writing Program. Health Studies, too, has provided a rich interdisciplinary community, and I thank Anna West for welcoming me into it. Laura McGrane, Raji Mohan, Lindsay Reckson, Debora Sherman, Gus Stadler, and Theresa Tensuan all played important roles in my becoming a literary scholar in the first place, and they warmly welcomed me back as a visiting faculty member. Marlen Rosas's friendship has enriched life on and off campus—I'm so glad we got off topic during that first meeting for coffee to talk about writing our book proposals. A fellow visitor on campus, Courtney Marshall, provided much needed camaraderie within academia and continues to do so from afar. I owe more than I can say to Kristin Lindgren, whose first-year writing seminar set me on the path to writing this book and who has been a friend, mentor, and colleague for over a decade.

I feel so fortunate to have found a community within nineteenth-century US literary studies that has made this work meaningful and sustainable. Thank you to Jessica Horvath Williams for bringing together disability studies scholars within our field and for feedback on material that appeared in the introduction and chapter 3. I am grateful to have been in conversation with Jess Cowing while developing chapter 4, and Vivian Delchamps provided fruitful discussions of disability literature along the way. I owe sincere thanks to Sarah Nance for being the most affirming reader and friend I could ask for and to Dan Couch for demystifying the publishing process and teaching my old dog a new trick. Sam Sommers deserves a special shout-out for championing me and my work so fiercely. Thank you, Clare Mullaney, for agreeing to meet with an eager undergraduate student applying to PhD programs and for remaining a friend ever since.

Much of this book was written in Philadelphia, where I have been lucky to be surrounded by many old and new friends. Though they've since moved away, Greer Cohen, Alex Eppler, Kasya O'Connor Grant, and Becky Suzuki all ensured that early research trips to the city were also joyful reunions. Since I moved to Philly, friends including Helen Farley, Aurora MacRae-Crerar, Vinayak Mathur, Cathy Mayer, and Lilly Mudge have provided both necessary distractions from and touching enthusiasm about this project. Matti Freiberg, Nora Howe, Haleh Kanani, and Michaela Ward have made Philly home. Thank you, Matt Goldberg, for sharing that home with me and for embracing the uncertainty of life in academia.

My family deserves special thanks. My father, Daryl Libow, died just as this project was beginning, but I know he would have read it cover to cover. I am grateful that my sister, Claudia Libow, has been my lifelong cheerleader and confidante. Finally, thank you to my mother, Beth Libow, who cared for my dog during research trips and cared for me in so many ways during the writing of this book.

Vigorous Reforms

Introduction

During the afternoon session of the first day of the June 1852 Woman's Rights Convention in West Chester, Pennsylvania, the discussion turned to health. After hearing remarks on the subject from expert speakers including Harriot Kezia Hunt, who would be awarded an honorary MD from the Women's Medical College of Pennsylvania the following year, and Elizabeth Blackwell, the first woman to earn a medical degree in the United States, Ernestine Rose took the floor. Rose, who would later be elected president of the Convention, declared that a "woman might be physician to herself and her children. But the medical schools are closed against her; she is denied the advantages granted to man, for obtaining knowledge of these things, more necessary if possible to her than to the other sex."[1] For Rose, health was not just one in a litany of disciplines to which women were denied access. Rather, she suggested that an understanding of health was vital to women's ability to oversee that which was already recognized as within their sphere of influence: their own bodies and those of the children in their care. Indeed, despite her decrying the exclusivity of "the medical schools," Rose was not interested in professionalized expertise alone. Unlike Hunt and Blackwell before her, she spoke from the perspective of the lay women in and beyond the Convention's audience for whom "knowledge of the art of healing" was both essential and elusive.[2]

Citing her own body as evidence of women's widespread deprivation of health knowledge, Rose turned to her audience, asking "Why am I, in the prime of life, in such feeble health?"[3] The explanation for her frailty, she insisted, was her lack of access to much-needed health information. "In my country," she lamented, "the laws of health are, comparatively speaking, kept in a nut shell. The girl must not exercise herself. It is not fashionable! She must not be seen in active life, it is not feminine. The boy may run, the girl must creep."[4] By locating health knowledge "in a nut shell," Rose implied that the information women needed in order to care for themselves and others was both significantly oversimplified and squirreled away by those in power. She acknowledged, too, that the "fashionable" nature of women's resultant weakness had significant consequences. Her juxtaposition of the boyish freedom to "run" and the restrained feminine "creep" signaled to the women in her audience both their imposed bodily limitations and the difficulty of their keeping pace with men in the "active" public sphere of the United States' physically and ideologically restrictive patriarchal culture.

As Rose's comments at the Convention make clear, both health knowledge and bodily health itself were important political tools that American women ardently sought and strategically deployed over the course of the nineteenth century. Largely shut out, as Rose notes, from formal medical education, women obtained information about their own and others' health by engaging in the study of physical education.[5] A domestic scientific discourse that combined exercise and hygienic homemaking with lessons in anatomy and physiology, the field was capacious enough to be applied to a variety of practices and contexts. "Physical education," the educator Almira Hart Lincoln Phelps explained in 1833, referred to "improvements which can be effected in the human frame and the senses by a proper system of discipline."[6] Indeed, the concept of "improvement" was integral to this feminized form of health knowledge and its adaptation to explicitly political ends. Throughout the nineteenth century, women writers drew insights from physical education to comment on political issues ranging from national expansion and enslavement to Indigenous sovereignty and immigration. If women could acquire the knowledge needed to enhance the human body, they reasoned, so too might they transform the institutions that exerted control over it.

Vigorous Reforms: Women Writers and the Politics of Health in the Nineteenth-Century United States traces how women writers leveraged the health knowledge they gained through physical education to intervene in contentious debates about sex, race, and citizenship. This book builds on a robust body of scholarship on illness and disability in nineteenth-century women's writing in order to illuminate health and ability as similarly vexed designations. From arguments that white women lacked the strength for rigorous education to the insistence that Black women's innate endurance fitted them for enslavement, physiological theories of sex and race constructed womanhood in relation to bodily capacity. At a time when human differences were often cast as biologically fixed, physical education equipped women to conceive of the body not as a static entity but instead as shaped by the various material circumstances over which they sought expanded influence. Tracing women's reform literature over the course of the century, I show how this view of health as a skill rather than an essential character impacted the formation both of white feminism and its violences and of Black and Indigenous feminist inquiries into health disparities.

Physical education was not only a way of responding to male-dominated medicine but was also a site of immense racial conflict among women reformers themselves. Far from a unified theory of the body and its management, physical education was a fragmented science and, as such, an equally dangerous and generative political tool. While white women reformers mobilized their health expertise against sexist social structures, they also weaponized it against women of color. As part of a larger health reform movement that "stitch[ed] nationalism to the individual white body," physical education equipped women to participate in political and social debates, and it also lent scientific authority to racist barriers to national belonging.[7] Indeed, many white writers suggested that their commitment to health was itself a sign of their racial superiority. At the same time, Black and Indigenous women articulated their own theories of health that they drew on to critique racist and colonial harms including those caused by white women reformers. Here I draw on Britt Rusert's framework of "fugitive science" and Julie Avril Minich's "radical health" to show how women of color reconstructed the terms of physical education and challenged the field's entrenched white nationalism.[8] As such, physical education was both a response to and an instrument of biopolitical processes such as enslavement and assimilation. For instance, while Margaret Fuller's 1844 travel narrative celebrated white girls' heightened capacity for physical development as an expression of settler-colonial power, Zitkala-Ša's (Yankton) exposed the debilitation caused by the use of physical education as a "civilizing" tool later in the century. Ultimately, *Vigorous Reforms* argues that physical education made ideas about health fundamental to the development of what we now call American feminism, including its internal conflicts.[9]

The Politics of Physical Education

Over the course of the nineteenth century, the meaning of "physical education" shifted significantly.[10] While antebellum manuals used the term to refer to an array of child-rearing and self-help activities that could be practiced by all women, the latter half of the century saw it coalesce into a distinct scientific field with exercise as its focal point. Whether taught by mothers or specially trained educators, though, "improvement" remained the goal. Physical education promised to cultivate superior bodies and, with them, elevated moral character.[11] The field was part of a broader biopolitical apparatus of health reform that included social movements including temperance and sexual hygiene, and that, Kyla Wazana Tompkins explains, posited that "the ideal citizen was to be made and remade via the quotidian practices of correct consumption, self-care, and sexual hygiene."[12] Physical education focused on the teaching of such practices, and this pedagogical orientation positioned health as firmly within the purview of women. By taking responsibility for shaping the ideal citizen, women could recast traditional domestic concerns as modern, scientific pursuits with significant consequences for the future of the nation.[13]

In the early nineteenth century, American women's physical education emerged as a domestic science taught in the home and classroom that circulated widely through advice manuals targeting mothers, caregivers, and teachers. In 1829, educator Catharine Beecher lamented white American women's ignorance of health. She insisted that young women be taught early on "the structure, the nature, and the laws of the body" so that they might "understand the operation of diet, air, exercise and modes of dress upon the human frame."[14] This, she suggested, was crucial not simply because it would allow women to become healthier themselves but also because it would equip them to instill this knowledge in others. "Is it not," she asked, "the business, the profession of a woman to guard the health and form the physical habits of the young?"[15] For Beecher and the physical education advocates who proliferated in her wake, knowledge of health would enable women to fulfill their obligation of caring for future generations.

In the ensuing decades, a number of women published domestic advice manuals that featured health instruction. Celebrated literary figures including Lydia Maria Child, Lydia Sigourney, and Catharine Maria Sedgwick all framed health as an important component of domestic knowledge. In *The Mother's Book* (1831), for instance, Child describes "a vigorous constitution" as "the greatest of earthly blessings" and explains the importance of mothers allowing their daughters to take "exercise in the open air."[16] Authors of these advice manuals tended to position themselves as maternal authority figures. The first manual by an American woman devoted exclusively to exercise instruction, *A Course of Calisthenics for Young Ladies, in Schools and Families* (1831), was published anonymously by "a mother." A few years later, a US edition of Irish writer Margaret King Moore's *Advice to Young Mothers on the Physical Education of Children* (1833) was attributed to "A Grandmother" on the title page. Professional teachers, too, played an important role in early physical education. Long before the establishment of specialized physical education normal schools, school teachers integrated health instruction into their curricula.[17] As early as 1800, Sarah Pierce required regular walking at the Litchfield Female Academy, and these lessons may have provided early inspiration for Beecher, who was one of her pupils.[18] Beecher's own advice manuals identified "schools," along with "homes" and "families" as her target audience. The anonymously authored *A Course of Calisthenics*, too, was "respectfully inscribed to mothers *and instructresses*."[19] As such, these volumes suggested that teachers' work in the schoolhouse mirrored the domestic instruction that took place at home.

Information about the body also circulated among women who attended "reform physiology" lectures hosted by female moral reform and physiological societies. Following the efforts of dietary reformer Sylvester Graham, lecturers warned the women in their audiences about the "solitary vice" of masturbation and its attendant health risks, and they also supplied them with a broader preventive health framework that included physical education's tenets of hygiene, diet, and exercise.[20] When the most famous of these experts, Mary Gove Nichols, published her *Lectures to Women on Anatomy and Physiology* in 1846, she stressed the importance of mothers' knowledge of health in particular. "Mothers, in their ignorance," she writes, "poison the very fountains of life and health."[21]

Women physical education advocates explicitly tied the improvements in health that they championed to the formation of an elevated national character. As Amy Kaplan has established in her landmark essay on "manifest domesticity," the domestic space was far from a "separate sphere" but was deeply enmeshed with public and political life under the banner of nationalism.[22] The application of this logic to health is evidenced in Catharine Maria Sedgwick's *Means and Ends: Or, Self-Training* (1842), in which the author insists that one's "moral and intellectual development" "depends mainly" on one's "physical being."[23] The cultivation of physical health, she explains, has far-reaching consequences, since "the wisdom and virtue manifested . . . from halls of legislation" is "formed, at home, by the mother, the first teacher."[24] The view of child-rearing as a civic duty that Linda Kerber calls eighteenth-century "Republican motherhood" appears in these later domestic manuals as a commitment to rearing a healthy population.[25]

By mid-century, women began to seek instruction beyond advice books, turning to male physicians for instruction in a field that became increasingly concerned with exercise in particular. While working as a teacher, writer Louisa May Alcott enrolled as a part-time student at Diocletian Lewis's celebrated Normal Institute for Physical Training, where she studied his widely popular "new gymnastics."[26] While Alcott's interest in health is evidenced by Jo March's propensity for outdoor exercise in *Little Women* (1868–69), her familiarity with physical education as a pedagogical tool is more prominently displayed in its sequel, *Little Men* (1871). In that novel, Jo and her husband open a school for boys where they prioritize "cultivating healthy bodies by much exercise," and it is this devotion to the next generation, rather than the development of her own health, that becomes the iconoclastic Jo's ultimate triumph—and proof of her domestication.[27]

The popularity of Lewis's institute paved the way for a host of other physical education normal schools that opened their doors in the 1880s. These schools ushered in a new model of physical education, as domesticity gave way to rigorous, specialized study and professional expertise. Physical education did, however, maintain its feminization. Dudley Allen Sargent, who directed the Normal School of Physical Training at Cambridge, Massachusetts (later the Sargent School of Physical Education), began by training only women and he espoused essentialist ideas that men's and women's respective capacities for exertion differed due to the physical demands of menstruation and reproduction.[28] Sargent and the many educators who followed his lead sought to maintain a separate professional sphere for women by insisting that girls required training distinct from boys, and that women teachers were especially suited to acquire knowledge of the female body.

Educators applied a similar logic to racial difference. Physical education normal schools differed from early exercise instruction in that they were interested in training Black as well as white women. In the late nineteenth and early twentieth centuries, many African American women attended the Sargent School of Physical Education, the Harvard University Summer School of Physical Training, and the Boston Normal School of Gymnastics (BNSG), where the playwright, poet, and birth control advocate Angelina Weld Grimké earned a degree.[29] That these teachers went on to teach at exclusively Black schools such as the Tuskegee Institute and Hampton Agricultural and Industrial School both created an opportunity to spread health knowledge within Black communities and reinforced the idea of race as biologically determined. For this new class of teachers, the determinism of physical education at once created new professional opportunities and dangerously used exercise to establish embodied scripts for social identities.[30]

This history of women's physical education has a rich history of its own. With the rise of women's studies in the latter half of the twentieth century, scholars turned to women's sports and exercise as part of a broader project of feminist historical recovery. This new wave of scholarship often registered exercise's pursuit of bodily control as inherently linked to feminist politics. Writing in 1978, sports historian Roberta Park remarked in an essay on nineteenth-century physical education that "one might be almost inclined to believe that modern woman's emancipation is intimately bound up with her athletic ability—or certainly with her physicality."[31] In 1990, Patricia Vertinsky similarly described early exercise enthusiasts as part of a broader, multigenerational movement of women who "rightly see health and physical expression as central to women's emancipation."[32] Vertinsky explicitly named this link between nineteenth-century women's exercise and late twentieth-century activism related to abortion and sexual violence by suggesting that early physical educators were "foreshadowing today's feminists" by arguing "that women must take control of their bodies."[33] Jan Todd, too, invoked the language of control in 1998, asserting that many women's "lives fundamentally changed" as a result of their newfound view of their bodies as "controllable."[34] These accounts appeared in the decades following the passage of Title IX, in which athletics (though unspecified in the law itself) became shorthand for combating sex-based discrimination in education. By suggesting that physical education was intrinsically and universally empowering for women, these historical studies echoed their primarily white, able-bodied subjects by leaving the link between health and feminism largely unquestioned.

More recent scholarship has addressed the role of race and sexuality in women's physical education. In her 2012 study of the first several decades of physical education's professionalization, Martha Verbrugge demonstrates how the field's emphasis on the materiality of the body gave rise to essentialist ideas about race, gender, and sexuality that codified these identities through "attitudes and habits."[35] As Verbrugge puts it, "analyzing physical education brings into new focus the tension between the nation's egalitarian ideals and record of discrimination."[36] Ava Purkiss has shown how Black women in the early twentieth century took up physical education as a public health measure and a strategy for promoting longevity and wellness among African Americans.[37] While these accounts tend to start at the end of the nineteenth century and focus primarily on developments in the twentieth, *Vigorous Reforms* extends such intersectional analysis of women's physical education to the antebellum United States in order to reconsider the effects of a (proto)feminist politics predicated on health. Whether taught in the home, the schoolroom, or the gymnasium, the various iterations of physical education that emerged over the course of the century shared a commitment to "improvement" that was deeply entangled with the project of American nationalism and thus had to negotiate the manifold exclusions and violences that project entailed. As a science of human transformation grounded in narrowly defined ideals, physical education carried both promise and profound limitations for women's reform efforts.

The Trouble with Health

One aim of this book is to demonstrate how physical education's keen attention to health offered an unstable foundation for reform. My method is grounded in Joan Burbick's assertion that "to read the narratives of the healthy body is to begin to understand the relationships of power and subordination that societies attempt to render invisible."[38] In this book, then, I use "health" to refer not merely to the experience of being "well" but also to what Jonathan Metzl describes as "a prescribed state and an ideological position."[39] Indeed, the ideology can have dangerous consequences for those deemed unhealthy, and throughout the nineteenth century, white women reformers instrumentalized what they perceived as the inferior bodies of women of color and disabled women in order to increase their own social and political authority.[40] White suffragists in particular rhetorically distanced themselves from disabled people and racialized minorities with whom they felt wrongfully affiliated by their shared disenfranchisement.[41] By staking their politics on narrowly constructed embodied ideals, many women reformers cast the political needs of those they deemed physically inferior and other as distinctly outside their movements' ultimate goals.

By many scholarly accounts, white feminist politics contributed to a devaluation of bodies perceived as impaired—including racialized bodies—with the rise of eugenics at the turn of the century. Eugenics, which sought to systematically eliminate supposedly "defective" human variations from the American body politic, found ready advocates in feminists such as Charlotte Perkins Gilman, Victoria Woodhull, and Margaret Sanger. Scholars have demonstrated how the eugenic emphasis on reproduction positioned white women as agents of racial nationalism, and how white women writers embraced this opportunity.[42] While chapter 5 shows how ideas about corporeal plasticity such as physical education existed alongside eugenic thinking, *Vigorous Reforms* also elaborates on a historical narrative that positions eugenics as the key juncture in the histories of women's activism and theories of human perfectibility. While physical education's theory of the body as malleable might seem to offer a redemptive counterpoint to eugenics' determinism, the two discourses shared a view of identity as biologically coded. As Kyla Schuller has shown, theories of corporeal pliability were deployed throughout the nineteenth century as a means of demarcating social groups and upholding hierarchies of human embodiment.[43] I propose that physical education, with its overt commitment to performing and producing a standardized American identity defined by whiteness and able-bodiedness, offers a crucial extension of the troubled relationship between white feminism and health.

Throughout this book, I follow scholars working in disability studies by interrogating the social value attached to health. Physical education illuminates corporeal designations beyond a disabled/able-bodied binary in part because it demands a preexisting degree of capacity in the pursuit of a state we might now call "fitness," which was often described as "vigor" in the nineteenth century. Just as disability is always contingently produced, as Rosemarie Garland-Thomson tells us, by material "misfits" between bodies and environments and, as Jasbir Puar asserts, by intersections with politically determined "assemblages of capacity and debility," so too is health highly fluid and contextual.[44] Social categories shift in situations where "health" can just as easily be defined by the ability to walk as by the ability to walk ten miles. As physical education developed over the course of the nineteenth century, women's expectations of their own and others' capabilities were constantly shifting, as were their efforts to cultivate bodies that could meet such standards.

Physical education also provides a window onto the interactions between discursive and material constructions of ability. Physical educators both theorized the body as disciplinable and actually disciplined pupils' bodies through scripted movements. As Sami Schalk and Jina B. Kim have shown, "discourses of disability . . . have real effects on women and people of color's body-minds."[45] Discourses of able-bodiedness such as physical education have similarly material consequences. Though prescriptive texts certainly may have benefited some women, they could also encourage or insist upon exhausting and injurious efforts. Furthermore, physical education advocates' construction of able-bodiedness as simultaneously desirable and universally achievable established health as a moral imperative, devaluing bodies that eschewed such standards. "Feminists," Susan Wendell argues, "have . . . criticized and worked to undo men's control of women's bodies, without undermining the myth that women can control their own bodies."[46] The "myth of control" over the body, she explains, pervades not only patriarchal culture, but also feminist movements that substitute patriarchal norms for an equally idealized body that is strong, capable, and controllable.[47] Julia Passanante Elman calls this strain of empowerment discourse "capacity feminism," noting how the conflation of physical strength with female empowerment leaves many women outside feminism's scope.⁴⁸ Indeed, many of the women whose writing I turn to in the chapters that follow documented their own embodied experiences of disability—whether temporary, remitting, or chronic. The tensions between these accounts and depictions of the idealized active body reveal the precarity of such corporeal criteria for feminist politics.

Women Writing Health

Vigorous Reforms draws on an expansive archive of physical education instruction that was disseminated through printed materials as well as school curricula, and it illuminates the health politics that women writers embedded in literary forms including travel narratives, sentimental novels, autobiography, and utopian fiction. As such, I demonstrate how women writers transposed and troubled the didactic discourse of physical education to a range of imaginative ends. Building on recent work by Josh Doty that demonstrates how theories of bodily change shaped literary expressions, I consider what literature reveals about the meanings attached to health.⁴⁹ That is, I argue that turning to writing by women reformers helps bring into focus the ideological functions of health.⁵⁰ While descriptions of and prescriptions for the actual practices nineteenth-century American women and girls performed are certainly crucial to understanding physical education's role in the development of women's activism, their literature illuminates the diverse symbolic functions of efforts to cultivate health. It also registers their ambivalence about and dissent from physical education's ideals. The chapters that follow thus track the development of physical education and its political implications over the hundred years preceding the Nineteenth Amendment's passage in 1920. This scope encompasses the formative decades of what we now call feminism in the United States, and it also reflects a period of immense changes to the composition of the American body politic.

In the early nineteenth century, the travel narrative offered women a genre through which to reflect on and critique what they saw as the dismal standards of female health in the still nascent United States. While scholars have shown how human maturation served as a metaphor for the young nation's national growth, chapter 1 considers narratives that posit a more literal connection. For many, the relative newness of the still growing nation offered an opportunity to intervene in female development through reforms in physical education. I begin with texts by British writers Frances Wright and Harriet Martineau, who sharply criticize the health habits of women and girls in the eastern US that they frame as detrimental to the nation but easily reformed, given the young country's malleability. I show how these travel narratives gave way to work by transcendentalist writer Margaret Fuller, who was born and raised in the New England culture that Wright and Martineau critique and who hoped national expansion might solve the problems they diagnosed. In *Summer on the Lakes, in 1843* (1844), which documents her trip to the western United States, Fuller's calls to reform girls' education there reveal the settler colonial underpinnings of such aspirations for white womanhood. This chapter thus sets the stage for the ensuing sections by establishing race and nation as foundational concerns for women health reformers.

Chapter 2 maps the concerns about national borders in the travel narrative genre onto a different domestic boundary: that of the home. This chapter centers on the debates about health labor across racial and class lines that played out on the bodies of the workers referred to as "domestics." These young women and girls were expected to learn about health and provide for others' physical well-being while laboring in environments that ultimately put their own health at risk. I begin by considering the work of domestic reformer Catharine Beecher, who routinely infantilized domestics by suggesting that they depended on their employers for both maternal guidance and health knowledge. From there, I consider critiques of this paradigm in what I call "the domestic's novel." Far from receiving an edifying physical education, the racialized Black and Irish domestics in novels by Catharine Maria Sedgwick and Harriet Wilson find that their health is routinely compromised—even deliberately harmed—in the same venues in which they work to provide for others' physical well-being. Racialized domestics, I argue, were revealed by reform-minded writers as precariously positioned health workers whose infantilized bodies were exploited rather than nurtured by the women who employed them.

While both free and enslaved Black women were often tasked with performing health labor on behalf of white families, chapter 3 considers how Black women also applied their health knowledge to radical, anti-racist ends. After publishing her narrative, *Incidents in the Life of a Slave Girl*, in 1861, abolitionist writer Harriet Jacobs traveled to Washington, DC, where she cared for refugees fleeing enslavement during the Civil War. Shortly after, she collaborated with her daughter, the domestic science educator Louisa Jacobs, to establish schools for Black children in Virginia and Georgia. In this chapter, I consider the discussions of health and child-rearing that appear in Jacobs's famous autobiography, and I recontextualize these alongside the ideas about Black health in her wartime dispatches to the abolitionist press and to Northern reform organizations. Jacobs, I argue, consistently frames her health aptitude not as the innate abilities of a "mammy" but rather as studied expertise in what she calls "the science of good management."[51] Furthermore, by transforming the health labor demanded of African American women by white enslavers and employers into practices of self- and community care, Jacobs's writing also subverts racist scientific claims of Black dependency on white supervision. Her approach to physical education locates caregiving networks beyond those accounted for in white women's reform discourse, highlighting an alternative, fugitive legacy of Black women and health science.

The book's two final chapters shift to the later part of the nineteenth century and to the institutional contexts in which women physical educators of that era exerted their influence. Chapter 4 centers on the Carlisle Indian Industrial School, where white educators adopted a comprehensive approach to physical education that shaped every aspect of student life. Their curriculum for girls combined domestic labor at the school and in white families' homes, Christian religious instruction, and choreographed exercise routines. In this chapter, I examine the highly scrutinized and regulated bodies of female students as sites of pedagogical debate that destabilized notions of "civilized" feminine comportment. My analysis turns on the work of three women educators: student newspaper supervisor Marianna Burgess; superintendent of Indian schools Estelle Reel; and oratory and music instructor Zitkala-Ša (Yankton). While white educators like Burgess and Reel insisted that their pedagogy corrected for deficiencies in their Indigenous pupils' bodies, Zitkala-Ša inverts this logic to illuminate the school's harmful effects. I show how social constructions of disability such as those expressed by Carlisle educators caused students' material debilitation. Ultimately, this chapter foregrounds Zitkala-Ša's exploration of labor, spirituality, and health in order to demonstrate how the imposition of physical education on communities deemed defective could actually produce the kinds of widespread physical impairments it purported to eradicate.

Chapter 5 extends this discussion of assimilation by considering the pedagogical treatment of immigrants at the turn of the twentieth century. By showing how physical education offered women a framework for confronting difference, I contribute a corollary to the established history of eugenic feminism's emphasis on reproduction by showing how white feminists expressed and negotiated eugenic impulses in their supervision of the children of immigrants. The first part of this chapter considers Jane Addams's Hull-House settlement in Chicago, where specially trained physical educators harnessed pupils' diverse backgrounds to forge a cosmopolitan approach to athletic activity. For Addams, wholesome physical activity offered an opportunity for intercultural exchange as well as an anchor to Old World traditions that she saw as more desirable alternatives to the indecent recreational activities of an emergent urban youth culture. I juxtapose this model with those outlined in the utopian novels of Charlotte Perkins Gilman, who briefly lived at Hull-House in the 1890s, and whose speculative fiction from the early 1910s combines that institution's emphasis on physical education for immigrants and their children with her own eugenic preoccupations. In Gilman's imagined and idealized worlds, normative physical education promises to standardize the foreign bodies that her novels figure as threats to national physiological ideals. By comparing Addams's and Gilman's theories, this chapter demonstrates how authority over physical education positioned women to respond to the perceived threat of a rapidly changing body politic.

Tracing this history brings into clearer focus the still vexed role of health in contemporary feminism. From reproductive justice to access to affordable health care, health activism remains urgent in the twenty-first century. At the same time, the banner term "health" can conflate such issues with the kinds of domestic practices that nineteenth-century women called physical education and thus risk supplanting policy change and political transformation with individual responsibility. As I demonstrate in the book's epilogue, physical education has been replaced today by the new domestic health science of wellness. While calisthenics have given way to spin classes, such commodities are nonetheless routinely branded as "radical" forms of self-care, echoing physical education's prior political connotations and maintaining its dangerous consequences. Audre Lorde's 1988 contention that "caring for myself is not self-indulgence, it is self-preservation and that is an act of political warfare" has been co-opted by a feminist-coded wellness industry that does little to address—and, indeed, often exacerbates—the drastic health disparities that continue to shape many American women's lives.[52] By historicizing the extent to which such contemporary domestic health practices are deeply inflected by ideas about gender, race, and national belonging, *Vigorous Reforms* makes clear that women writers have long wielded their health knowledge to political ends—for better and for worse.

CHAPTER ONE

The Future of White Womanhood in Young America

In her 1819 pamphlet presented before the New York legislature, *A Plan for Improving Female Education*, Emma Willard calls for a publicly funded seminary for young women that will "bring its subjects to the perfection of their moral, intellectual, and physical nature."[1] In her proposal, which includes provisions for "exercise . . . needful to the health . . . of youth" in the form of supervised dancing, Willard insists that "youth . . . should be wholly devoted to improvement" for all pupils.[2] To conclude her pamphlet, Willard reminds her legislative audience that it is not only prospective students whose development is at stake, but also that of the young nation. She declares the cause of female education a matter of "national glory" and an intervention in an otherwise disappointing history of gender politics.[3] "Where," she asks, "is that wise and heroic country, which has considered, that [women's] rights are sacred, though we cannot defend them? That tho' [sic] a weaker, we are an essential part of the body politic, whose corruption or improvement must affect the whole?"[4] Though she laments that "history shows not that [the] country" regards women's "improvement" as essential to its own, she optimistically adds that "anticipation does."[5] For Willard, the progressive spirit of the still young United States is uniquely conducive to the reforms she seeks.

In the pamphlet's final line, Willard clarifies how improving women's education will benefit the still evolving nation. "Who knows," she asks, "how great and good a race of men, may yet arise from the forming hand of mothers, enlightened by the bounty of that beloved country, — to defend her liberties, — to plan her future improvement — and to raise her to unparalleled glory?"[6] If given ample opportunity for improvement, she suggests, female students might go on to "raise" a superior class of men, who in turn will implement further reforms and allow the nation to progress beyond its predecessors.

The ambiguous subject of this concluding call for *"her* improvement" reflects Willard's and other women reformers' belief in the reciprocal relationship between the development of young women and that of the young United States. Sari Edelstein has shown how "age ideology narrativize[d] nationalist projects" for many late eighteenth- and early nineteenth-century American writers who invoked human development as a metaphor for the country's maturation.[7] The relationship between the two could also be quite literal. In this chapter, I show how antebellum women writers' travel narratives constructed the changing character and expanding borders of the new nation as opportunities to intervene in the development of the female population by increasing girls' access to physical education. By their assessments, the youthful malleability of what historians have called the "adolescent" nineteenth-century United States meant that its national norms had not yet solidified, making it ripe for reform.[8] They argued that as the nation changed, so too might its practices of educating girls, and that women who received the benefits of a healthful youth would in turn be better equipped to sustain and contribute to this continued progress.

This tendency among women writers to position the United States' newness as grounds for transformation is distinct from, but partly concurrent with, the literary cadre of male authors who referred to themselves as "Young Americans." From 1837 to the mid-1850s, writers including John O'Sullivan, Evert Duyckinck, Cornelius Matthews, Nathaniel Hawthorne, and Walt Whitman sought to channel the spirit of the American Revolution by articulating a vision of the national future that distinguished it from other countries and fulfilled the ideals of the nation's founders.[9] While these literary nationalists saw themselves as heralding a new generation of Americans, the women writers I turn to in this chapter staked their hopes for the nation on an even younger set: girls. Rather than present *themselves* as embodiments of the national future, they turned their attention to the next generation, advocating for educational reforms of which health was a central component. Further contrary to the brand of literary nationalism practiced by the Young Americans, not all of the women examined in this chapter were, in fact, Americans. Accounts by British writers such as Frances Wright and Harriet Martineau show that this progressive view of a nation that many Americans hoped could be a site of gender progress appealed to reformers across the Atlantic as well.

The travel accounts by Wright, Martineau, and the American transcendentalist Margaret Fuller that I assess here characterize the United States as a young nation still in development, and all three apply their knowledge of health to imagine the country's future potential. Lila Marz Harper has argued that the genre of the travel narrative offered a unique opportunity for scientific-minded women to participate in male-dominated discourses, and the texts I examine in this chapter establish human health as among the scientific fields to which they contributed.[10] In each of these narratives, the writers arrive in locales where they expect to find progressive gender politics and are dismayed to discover the state of girls' and women's health there. Each insists that the new environment not only is ripe for innovations in female physical education but also requires such reforms in order to achieve its ideals. I begin with Wright's *Views of Society and Manners in America* (1821) and Martineau's *Society in America* (1837), both of which present improvements in female health as sorely needed reforms that will allow the new nation to enact the principles of equality upon which it was founded. I then turn to Fuller's account of the newly established state of Michigan in *Summer on the Lakes, in 1843* (1844). In this text, Fuller adopts a stance similar to her British predecessors in her assessment of settler girls' health, but her treatment of their Indigenous counterparts lays bare the nationalistic foundations of tethering health reform to colonized land.

Frances Wright, Republicanism, and Women's Health

In 1818, Wright, a young Scottish woman, realized her dream of visiting the United States, a new nation that she hoped would give rise to new social formations. Wright, who would famously go on to lecture before "promiscuous audiences" of both men and women on reform issues from free thought to abolition, published observations from her first journeys to the United States in *Views of Society and Manners in America* (1821). The book is organized as a series of letters addressed "to a friend in England" and reflects Wright's "excessive optimism about the American project" and the potentially elevated status of women within it.[11] Since its initial publication, critics have derided *Views* for its naïvely celebratory outlook on the United States. In 1828, the American author James Fenimore Cooper dismissed it as "nauseous flattery."[12] More recently, historian Gail Bederman has argued that Wright's idealism regarding the new nation distorted her view of its failings, leading her to "misrecognize[] slavery" as a British-influenced anomaly in an otherwise prefect nation rather than as one of the United States' foundational institutions.[13] Much scholarship on Wright has thus focused primarily on her eventual attempt to eradicate what she saw as this blemish on American society through the failed utopian Nashoba Community as well as on her status as a radical free thought lecturer.[14] As these accounts rightly demonstrate, *Views* was Wright's entrée into the reform circles where she would soon become known, but it was also an important text in its own right, establishing the sociological travel narrative as a tool that white women could employ to critique various aspects of US culture during the first half of the nineteenth century.[15] To the twenty-three-year-old Wright who authored *Views*, the United States was a "young and vigorous world"—at once new and healthy.[16] As such, she imbued it with immense potential for further growth. A healthy young America, she suggested, was not simply a metaphor for a well-governed society. On the contrary, she proposed that the health of the population was essential to the new republic's ongoing progress. Channeling the opening line of John Locke's *Some Thoughts Concerning Education* (1693), which begins "A Sound Mind in a sound Body," Wright declares in *Views* that "to invigorate the body is to invigorate the mind, and Heaven knows that the weaker sex have much cause to be rendered strong in both."[17] The previously neglected health of women, she suggested, was thus crucial to the nation's realizing its full potential.

The political sensibilities Wright exhibits in *Views* were significantly shaped by her relationships with late eighteenth-century Scottish intellectuals. Indeed, Jane Rendell argues that her travel narrative might "be read as a product of the late—very late—years of the Scottish Enlightenment."[18] Orphaned at age two and reared by Tory grandparents, Wright fled this conservative environment when she turned eighteen and went to live with her uncle, James Mylne, a moral philosophy professor at the University of Glasgow, and his wife, Agnes. There, she was exposed to an intellectual milieu that spurred her interest in republicanism. Among her new social set was Robina Craig Millar, the "friend in England" to whom she addresses the letters that comprise *Views*. Millar was the daughter-in-law of the Scottish philosopher and historian John Millar. As Rendell has observed, the sociological analysis in *Views* was almost certainly influenced by John Millar's *Observations Concerning the Distinction of Ranks in Society* (1771), which begins with a chapter entitled "Of the Rank and Condition of Women in Different Ages."[19] Robina Craig Millar's own prominent father, William Cullen, a professor of medicine at the University of Edinburgh, also influenced Wright. One of Cullen's former students was the preeminent American physician and signer of the Declaration of Independence, Benjamin Rush.[20] Rush became a close friend of Millar's, having warmly welcomed her and her husband when they traveled to the United States in 1795. Though Millar ultimately returned to Scotland after her husband's sudden death, she maintained her correspondence with Rush until his own passing in 1813—the same year that Wright joined her social circles.[21]

Upon arriving in the US, Wright lamented Rush's having died before she made her voyage. In *Views*, she mourns the "late Dr. Rush" to Millar, reflecting that his passing "makes even the young pause to ruminate on the swift wings of time, when they find the path of life forsaken by those whom the heart has been taught to venerate."[22] More than mere respect for a mutual friend, Wright ardently admired Rush's theories. The republicanism Wright encountered among her relatives' set was still seen as radical within the United Kingdom, but it was ultimately an "anachronistic, 1790s version of Anglo-American republicanism."[23] Rush in particular seems to have influenced both her advocacy for improvements in women's education and her attention to the role of health within a republic. As Sari Altschuler has demonstrated, Rush and his contemporaries "hoped that republican health would provide a more solid and salubrious basis for the republican polity."[24] Wright, too, adopted this view, portraying citizen health as politically necessary. She also shared with Rush what Justine S. Murison identifies as an early republican paradox, wherein one's psychological state was seen as simultaneously a qualification for and a product of inclusion within the American political order. For Wright, this "circular psychological problem" manifested in women's lack of physical health.[25] She suggests that elevating their health would both solidify women's status within the nation and bolster the republic itself.

Throughout *Views*, Wright proposes that the overall American population is healthier than that of Europe. She insists, for instance, that "the climate of this continent . . . seems to be peculiarly healthy, and highly favourable to the growth of the human figure."[26] "I imagine," she continues, "there are more instances of extraordinary longevity in these states, than you could find in any part of Europe."[27] Wright portrays the United States as a nation of physically active citizens who thoroughly embrace and benefit from the environment they inhabit. She draws a quote from British lieutenant Francis Hall's *Travels in Canada, and the United States, in 1816 and 1817* (1818) to argue that the "plentiful, but simple food, a health climate, [and] constant exercise in the open air" observed in Americans "account for the differing stature between Europeans and Americans."[28] She explains that the American farmer is "universally" "exposed to air and exercise" and produces "numerous offspring, whose nerves are braced by exercise, and their minds invigorated by liberty."[29] By her account, the United States is an ideal environment for human development, and this healthful growth is crucial to the republic's functionality. She argues that "it is the union of bodily and mental vigor in the male population of America which imparts to it that peculiar energy of character" that she associates with a republicanism that she ultimately hopes to extend to the nation's women.[30]

Strangely, although she deems both American health and gender politics superior to European standards, she nonetheless finds the women remain generally "enervated in soul and body" and thus calls for increased attention to their physical education.[31] "I often lament," she writes, "that in the rearing of women, so little attention should be commonly paid to the exercise of the bodily organs."[32] For Wright, the problem of female frailty is uniquely urgent within the US context. This is both because American women's bodies are notably inferior to their male counterparts, who she claims have surpassed Europeans in health and, more importantly, because a representative democracy relies on the character of all of its citizens. Wright draws this view of women's education from Rush, quoting his 1786 treatise *On the Mode of Education Proper in a Republic*: "I am sensible that our women must concur in all our plans of education for young men, or no laws will ever render them effectual . . . the obligations of patriotism should be inculcated upon them."[33] Wright fears that Rush's call has not been heeded, and that American women remain "deficient" in their understanding of republicanism. "They love their country, and are proud of it," she writes of these women, but only because "it *is* their country," while "their husbands love and are proud of it because it is free and well-governed."[34] Only when women's patriotic sensibilities become "enlightened" enough to mirror those of their male counterparts "will the national character . . . be yet more marked than it is at present."[35]

Wright frames physical health as directly conducive to such politically requisite mental capacity. Women, she suggests, cannot display "a vigorous intellect" because "it is broken down by sufferings, bodily and mental."[36] "To invigorate the character," and achieve moral parity with American men, she explains, "the body also must be trained to wholesome exercise"—women must learn "to excel in the race, to hit a mark, [and] to swim."[37] Such exercise, she promises, will "impart vigor to [women's] frames and independence to their minds."[38] Here Wright channels the British writer Mary Wollstonecraft's *A Vindication of the Rights of Woman: With Strictures on Political and Moral Subjects* (1793), in which she proposes that "by being allowed to take the same exercise as boys, not only during infancy, but youth," "women would acquire" the "strength of body" "sufficient to enable them to earn their own subsistence, the true definition of independence."[39] When Wright refers to "independence," however, she refers neither to economic self-sufficiency nor to later feminist formulations of an autonomous subject. Rather, she alludes to the spirit of republicanism that she sees as having been the impetus for American independence. As Lisa Pace Vetter has shown, Wright believed that only through universal education could the United States maintain the egalitarianism on which it was presumably founded.[40] Writing in 1821, Wright finds that the "cooperation of the sexes" that she believes prevailed during the American Revolution has faltered because the current generation of women has been educated "too much after the European manner."[41] She writes that in order for the nation "to preserve in her sons the energy of freemen and patriots, she must strengthen that energy in her daughters."[42] Regaining the bodily "energy" that has been "broken down" in American women, she suggests, might help restore this republican ideal.

Importantly, Wright portrays these "daughters" as future mothers when she imagines that as a result of an improved educational system, "a new race, nurtured under the watchful eye of judicious mothers, and from them imbibing, in tender youth, the feelings of generous liberty and ardent patriotism."[43] Wright frames women's expanded political education as vital to their maternal responsibilities and, as such, advocates for what Linda Kerber calls "Republican Motherhood."[44] Wright would have encountered this sentiment in Rush's treatise on education, in which he reminds readers that "the first impressions upon the minds of children are generally derived from the women. Of how much consequence, therefore, is it in a republic, that they should think justly upon the great subject of liberty and government!"[45] Wright builds on this assertion, making clear that such an emphasis on the character that women might cultivate through physical activity is particularly suited to the context of a nation "where a mother is charged with the formation of an infant mind that is to be called in future to judge of the laws and support the liberties of the republic."[46]

Wright concludes her letter on education in *Views* apologetically. "But I have dwelt enough upon this subject," she signs off, "and you will, perhaps apprehend that I am about to subjoin a Utopian plan of national education: no, I leave this to the Republic herself; and, wishing all success to her endeavours, I bid you farewell."[47] However, Wright did believe that such a "Utopian plan" would be needed in order to bring about improvements in women's health. In *Views*, she is optimistic that the character of women will improve "as their education shall become, more and more, the concern of the state," and indeed Wright would go on to advocate for a nationwide system of public education.[48] This she modeled after the schools at Robert Owen's New Harmony community, where Wright was a frequent resident throughout 1824. In an 1829 lecture, Wright appealed to classical republicanism, insisting that the United States should have "what Sparta had—a national education," but also, having been shaped by Enlightenment sensibilities, "what Sparta, in many respects, had not—a rational education."[49] Notably, the classical model that Wright hoped to elevate was forged not only "at the public board" but also "in the gymnasium."[50] She aspired for all children, including girls, to have "the same advantages, mental, moral, and physical" and that the formation of such a "common condition" would help give rise to the ideal republic she had crossed the Atlantic hoping to find.[51]

Harriet Martineau and the Consequences of American Apathy

By Harriet Martineau's assessments, the decade following Wright's *Views* saw few of the reforms in female education that she championed. In 1834, Martineau commenced a two-year journey throughout the United States that she documented in the multivolume tract *Society in America* (1837) (published in three volumes in England and two in the United States) and the shorter *Retrospect of Western Travel* (1838).[52] Martineau shared Wright's enthusiasm about America's relative youth, but she was far more critical of the country than her predecessor. Martineau, who had found recent success adapting theories of political economy into fictional narratives in her nine-volume *Illustrations of Political Economy* (1834), subscribed to the ideas about demography espoused by her friend, the English economist Thomas Robert Malthus. In *An Essay on the Principle of Population* (1798), Malthus argued that the differential rates of increase in a society's population and its food production levels led to inevitable poverty and "children [who] are sickly from insufficient food."[53] To address this problem, he controversially called for repealing the British Poor Laws that granted government relief to those living in poverty, claiming this would provide a "positive check" to the population by disincentivizing the poor from having large families.[54] In an 1803 revision of his original essay, Malthus also added "moral restraint" from reproduction as a possible preventive check against population growth. While Martineau's Malthusian ideas about demography and population growth are not the focus of her travel narratives, his concerns about population health certainly color her observations. Over the course of her travels, she repeatedly takes note of the American population's substandard health as well as its reciprocal relationship to the morality of its citizens.

Throughout *Society*, Martineau assesses the character of the United States using its own standard, the Declaration of Independence. She routinely points out the nation's failure to enact the democratic notions articulated therein, with slavery the clearest illustration of its unfulfilled ideals. She portrays the American population as "a young and inexperienced people" and regards their national failings as expressions of an adolescent folly that she hopes they will collectively outgrow.[55] In *Society* she reminds European readers that "it must be remembered how young the society is; how far it has already gone beyond most other countries."[56] As Ted Hovet argues, Martineau believed that the young country "contained the seeds of genuine reform, revision, and even revolution in social and political sphere," even if these had not yet come to fruition.[57] Her distinct version of American exceptionalism was premised on her belief that the young nation's age made its norms malleable and left its future still undecided.

While scholars have often compared Martineau's travelogue to British novelist Frances Trollope's *Domestic Manners of the Americans* (1832) and French diplomat Alexis de Tocqueville's *Democracy in America* (1835 and 1840), reading Martineau's text alongside Wright's illuminates her interest in women's health as a tool of political reform.[58] Martineau's professional correspondence reveals that she intended for "the chapters on Woman" in *Society* to have significant political impact on both sides of the Atlantic. She hoped, she told her editor, that her account would "expose [woman's] whole state, from her bad nursery training to her insulted wifehood in palaces, & her wretchedness in prostitution."[59] Indeed, in *Society*, Martineau declares that "woman's intellect is confined, her morals crushed, her health ruined, her weaknesses encouraged, and her strength punished" by American social norms.[60] Like Wright, she asserts that improving women's health is prerequisite to the US enacting its founding principles. By limiting women's opportunities, rights, and protections, Martineau argues, "the Americans have, in the treatment of women," she declares, "fallen below, not only their own democratic principles, but the practice of some parts of the Old World."[61] She presents the United States' treatment of women as a failure of the nation not only to meet its own espoused ideals but also to fulfill the promise of its youth and progress beyond older nations.

Martineau saw reforming women's education as an urgent need. In one of her earliest published works, an anonymous 1823 essay in the *Monthly Repository* entitled "On Female Education," she argues that British women's apparent inferiority is a product not of any "natural deficiency of power" but rather of their limited opportunities to "employ their faculties" and develop them to the fullest extent.[62] She laments that women are left only to the "peculiar duties" of "household occupations."[63] While she doesn't deny the importance of proper training in domestic labor, she argues that this knowledge is "easily acquired" and thus leaves room to expand women's tutelage to "nobler" fields of study as well.[64] Years later, in *Society*, Martineau echoes Wright's claim that women in the United States are educated "too much after the European manner" when she writes that "female education in America is much what it is in England," and is therefore both unsatisfactory and incongruous with the standards of equality by which Martineau judges the nation.[65] Rather than prepare women to assume parity with their male counterparts, Martineau argues, the lessons they receive "serve to fill up time, to occupy attention harmlessly, to improve conversation, and to make women something like companions to their husbands, and able to teach their children somewhat."[66] She suggests that women's education does little more than improve their performance of the domestic roles of wife and mother.

Rather than reiterate Wright's championing of healthful republican motherhood, though, Martineau insists that this emphasis on women's domestic responsibilities is itself detrimental to their health. Her primary objection is that American women spend too much time indoors and that they are oblivious to the threat this poses to them. She reports, "The ladies plead that they have much exercise within doors, about their household occupations."[67] Dismayed by this popular belief, Martineau notes that "except making beds, rubbing tables, and romping with children, I know of no household occupations which involve much exercise."[68] She also argues that therapeutic "walking" in "fresh air" is necessary to offset the bodily "weariness" that the most physically demanding chores produce.[69] Here Martineau establishes her own superior knowledge of health, framing what she describes as "apathy on the subject of health" as a distinctly American quality.[70] As "proof of the badness of the system of non-exercising," Martineau reports that "distortion of the spine is even more common among women in America than in Europe."[71] As concerning evidence, she cites physicians who "declare that the difficulty is to find in boarding-schools a spine that is perfectly straight."[72] This deficiency in young girls, she insists, is clearly a product of the habits and attitudes they've inherited from their American mothers. She observes that "Invalids are remarkably uncomplaining and unalarmed; and their friends talk of their having 'a weak breast,' and 'delicate lungs,' with little more seriousness than the English use in speaking of a common cold."[73] She recalls, too, the "extremest [sic] case" she encountered: "a lady, who declared, with complacency, that she could not walk a mile."[74] American women, she suggests, are not only inactive, but complacently so. Martineau's view of this as a severe incapacity—and a concerning illustration of "apathy"—is underscored by an earlier scene in *Society* in which she makes clear that walking is both a priority and a skill among British women. She recalls that her own lengthy walks of up to five miles were "much to the surprise of some persons, who were not aware how English ladies can walk."[75] Though she claims that neither the United States nor England has achieved a satisfactory system of women's education, Martineau's discussion of women's health knowledge suggests that American education has not simply failed to progress beyond that of England, but is actually far inferior in its neglect of girls' physicality.

According to Martineau, the prevalence of female frailty has serious consequences for the nation's moral standards. In *How to Observe: Morals and Manners* (1838), the methodological guide she published the year following *Society in America*, Martineau explains to her aspiring sociologist readers that "the Health of a community is an almost unfailing index of its morals," and she cites the United States as a prime example of a nation in which "the common deficiency of health produces moral effects which must strike the most careless traveler."[76] Indeed, throughout *Society*, she repeatedly asserts that "the morals of women are crushed" by the same limited sphere that she argues impairs their health.[77] She explains that the possession of a "conscience" is "virtually prohibited to beings who, like the American women, have scarcely any objects in life proposed to them."[78] She attributes women's lack of moral conscience to the same "power, custom, and education" that she elsewhere blames for their depleted health.[79]

Without moral strength, Martineau insists, women are ill equipped to contribute to the reform efforts she views as imperative to America's reaching its full potential, and especially to the abolition movement. In the concluding chapter of *Society*, she argues that the immorality exhibited by the persistence of slavery cannot be a product of America's republican "political organization," but must instead be attributed to "a host of other influences," which she elsewhere makes clear include health.[80]

Just as she deems the majority of American women's morals "crushed," so too does she disdain the "efforts made to crush the actions of women who . . . used their human powers in the abolition question."[81] She recalls a conversation with an American "lady" who asks her, "do you not think it a pity that so much is said on slavery just now?"[82] When Martineau replies that, on the contrary, she finds it "necessary and natural" to discuss the subject, the woman concedes that, though slavery may be a matter of "great consequence," she ultimately determines that "it is no business of ours; of us women, at all events."[83] Wary of American women's faltering morals, Martineau retorts, "I thought you considered yourself a Christian," to which the woman replies, seemingly weary with this position, "So I do. You will say that Christians should help sufferers, whoever and wherever they may be. But not women, in all cases, surely."[84] When Martineau pushes her to clarify, "she could only reply that she thought women should confine themselves to doing what could be done at home."[85] Unable to fathom "what in the world has . . . womanhood to do with" one's sense of moral obligation, Martineau is once again dismayed by American women's being trained exclusively for domestic responsibilities, though here she clarifies the stakes of such mistreatment.[86] American women's interrelated physical and moral failings are not only evidence of the nation's failure to meet its republican ideals but also perhaps one of its causes. She argues that women's apathy toward their own material health not only parallels but actually begets the harm to the national body politic perpetuated by their passive stance on a subject as urgent as abolition.

At the same time, Martineau insists that it is not too late to rehabilitate both American women's bodies and the nation's moral health. In *How to Observe*, she declares that "the best influence upon the morals of the American nation would be such as might improve their health."[87] In *Society*, Martineau offers concrete suggestions to this end. While "the common excuse for the deficient activity and lack of fresh air is the climate," she reports that "those who wish for health and know how to seek it, contrive to walk in summer very early in the morning; like residents in India. The mornings of the sultry months are perfectly delicious; and there is no excuse for neglect of exercise while they last."[88] She worries especially that schoolgirls are not taking adequate exercise. "Instead of sitting still all through the hot weather," she proposes, "and all through the cold weather, they had better exercise their limbs during some portion of the day, and lie down during the most sultry hours; and in the winter, avail themselves of every opportunity for active employment." "If they would do this," she hopes, "it is not to be conceived that the next generation would be distinguished as the present is for its spare forms and pallid complexions."[89] She proposes that adjusting their habits will give rise to a new model of female embodiment marked by health rather than impairment.

Another excuse for American women's inactivity, "the absence of convenient and pretty walks in and about the cities," she sees as merely a growing pain for the young nation.[90] Although "it is one of the misfortunes of a new country that its cities have environs which are little tempting for walking," she "trust[s]" that these "will be supplied in time."[91] She bolsters this point by highlighting an exception to the trend of female frailty: "a troop of rosy, graceful girls, and active women" in Stockbridge, Massachusetts, where "much pedestrian exercise . . . is accomplished."[92] If these women and girls are able to pursue exercise, Martineau reasons, then clearly the American environment is not to blame. "The way to have good country walks provided," she argues, "is to wish for them. When the whole female society of America shall be as fond of exercise, as highly principled with regard to it, as the Stockbridge ladies, the facilities will be furnished."[93] She promises that all of these provisions will have positive moral effects. She recalls an exchange with "a most liberal-minded clergyman" who sought her advice on how Americans might recapture the "strong religious sensibility" of the Pilgrims.[94] Martineau recommends, among other prescriptions, "more rational promotion of health, by living according to the laws of nature, which ordain bodily exercise and mental refreshment."[95]

By characterizing the lack of exercise opportunity as a "misfortune[] of a new country," Martineau implies that the US population will eventually improve in health, a transformation that will lead to increased morality. Lauren M. E. Goodlad calls this Martineau's "romance of improvement," which figures social reform "as a distant outcome, providentially sanctioned but actuated romantically through self-development."[96] Indeed, what Martineau calls "self-perfection" offers her a metaphor for explaining the young nation's moral failings.[97] In *Society*, she describes the United States as a miseducated woman, not unlike the female residents whose narrow training she elsewhere critiques. She suggests that "if America had been as free, from the beginning, in all respects, as a young country ought to be, — free to run her natural course of prosperity," the nation might have evaded the "original infection" of slavery that has "afflicted" it.[98] Just as the influences of European education limit women's health, so too does the inheritance — or, to use her medical metaphor, transmission — of slavery impair the republic. Ever invested in America's youth, though, Martineau does still hope that while "the old world will still be long in getting above its bad institutions," the new nation might "start afresh" and become "the first to show" the political and economic value of democratic ideals articulated during its founding.[99] Indeed, Martineau concludes *Society* by reminding readers once again of the young nation's great potential, writing that "American society itself constitutes but the first pages of a great book of events, into whose progress we can see but a little way; and that but dimly. It is too soon yet to theorize; much too soon to speak of conclusions even as to the present entire state of this great nation."[100] For Martineau, the US remains a work in progress, and improving women's physical and moral health might help rewrite its national story.

Martineau's optimistic view of Americans' potential is evident in her recollections of the transcendentalist writer Margaret Fuller. In her *Autobiography* (1877), Martineau recalls that upon *Society's* publication, the high-minded Fuller wrote to her critiquing the volume's emphasis on abolition and disparaging "the anti-slavery subject as simply a low and disagreeable one."¹⁰¹ Martineau, of course, disagreed with Fuller's assessment, which echoed that of the woman she debated in *Society*. However, she interpreted the young writer's statement as indicative of social rather than individual failings. After the younger woman's untimely death years later, Martineau expressed her confidence that Fuller, who spent the last years of her life in Europe, was likely "better aware . . . that the struggle for the personal liberty of millions in her native republic ought to have had more of her sympathy."¹⁰² Martineau observed her "intimate friend" sociologically, and "regard[ed] [Fuller's] American life as a reflexion [sic] . . . of the prevalent social spirit of her time and place."¹⁰³

Fuller herself took a remarkably similar view of her own character, and conveyed this self-perception to Martineau during their initial meeting in Boston in 1835. Martineau later recalled, "she told me what danger she had been in from the training her father had given her, and the encouragement to pedantry and rudeness which she derived from the circumstances of her youth."¹⁰⁴ Indeed, Fuller, who hoped Martineau might become an "intellectual guide" who would "comprehend [her] wholly, mentally and morally," shared the view articulated in *Society* that American women's deficient education compromised their interrelated physical and moral health—including her own.¹⁰⁵

National and Bodily Development in Margaret Fuller's *Summer on the Lakes*

Throughout the early 1840s, Fuller reflected on the education she received in the New England milieu that both Wright and Martineau critiqued. Fuller, who experienced chronic migraines and back pain throughout her life, was convinced that her ongoing impairments were the product of an overly sedentary youth and that the injurious system of educating American girls was in urgent need of reform. Fuller was not alone in this assessment, and she wrote about the physical education reform efforts of other American women such as Catharine Beecher and Catharine Maria Sedgwick for the *New-York Tribune*.¹⁰⁶ The ideas espoused by such physical education advocates offered Fuller an opportunity to translate transcendentalism's emphasis on self-cultivation into a broader apparatus of social reform.¹⁰⁷ Scholars have long recognized the centrality of embodiment to Fuller's feminist strain of transcendentalism, which, as C. Michael Hurst puts it, "sutures the body and mind back together."¹⁰⁸ If the body is, as Fuller claims in her most famous work, *Woman in the Nineteenth Century* (1845), "the abode and organ of the soul," then proper education requires cultivation of the corporeal as well as spiritual elements of the individual.[109]

Much as Wright and Martineau saw the newness of the United States as an opportunity to implement such reforms, Fuller turned her attention to the newly acquired Great Lakes, hoping that this younger extension of the nation might give rise to a new model of female physical education. In her account of her westward journey, *Summer on the Lakes, in 1843* (1844), she echoes her British predecessors' dismay and is aghast to find that the New England pedagogical methods she deems dangerous prevail among Illinois farm communities. As Susan L. Roberson has shown, "writing about travel to the West gave writers space to think about the nation and the direction it was taking," and for Fuller, this direction depended largely on improving the health of settler girls.[110] Her calls for health reform in the West ultimately reveal the settler colonial underpinnings of such aspirations for white womanhood by figuring Indigenous girls' deterioration and erasure from the American landscape as a prerequisite for white female health and, by extension, national progress.

Though a young Fuller told Martineau that her education impaired her character, Martineau's own writing may have helped illuminate her attention to its health effects. She would have read the critique of Amos Bronson Alcott's Temple School that Martineau includes in *Society*, which was published just as Fuller left her post as a teacher at that very school. In her account, Martineau criticizes Alcott's "outrageous" curriculum, which she was sure would "irreparably injure" students "morally as well as physically" through its "neglect of bodily exercises and over-excitement of brain."[111] Though Fuller adopted Alcott's view of the child as what she called a uniquely "still plastic human being," she too criticized his lack of attention to the body.[112] In her journal, she recorded a conversation in which she told him "you do not understand the reaction of matter on spirit."[113]

Unlike her fellow transcendentalist Henry David Thoreau, who deemed physical self-improvement "the whole duty of man" and a lifelong pursuit, Fuller believed that health was determined in youth.[114] She was convinced that "much of [her] life was devoured in the bud" and, at age thirty-seven, lamented, "firm health I see I cannot have. It is too late."[115] Like Wright, Fuller's ideas about health were influenced by Locke. In addition to invoking his famous maxim in *Woman*, writing that "only in a strong and clean body can the soul do its message fitly," she heeded his claims in *Some Thoughts Concerning Education* (1693) regarding the "lasting Consequences" of the "Impressions of our tender Infancies."[116] Elaborating on Locke's view of childhood as formative, Jean-Jacques Rousseau's *Émile; or, On Education* (1762), which Fuller read as a teenager, articulates a theory of sexual development that further clarifies youth's significance to Fuller's feminist project. Children, he proposes, lack sexual distinction. He explains that "up to the nubile age children of the two sexes have nothing apparent to distinguish them: the same visage, the same figure, the same complexion, the same voice. Everything is equal: girls are children, boys are children, the same name suffices."[117] By marking children as presexual, Rousseau provides a basis for Fuller's turn to youth as an ideal site of intervention. If what Fuller describes as the "nervous susceptibility" of women's "physical structure" is, as she claims, produced by educational norms, then such a corrective must occur as early as possible in order to minimize sex-based physical differences in adults. Youth therefore offered her a crucial but fleeting opportunity to intervene in female development.

In her unpublished "Autobiographical Romance," which she began in 1840, Fuller reflects on what she calls the "Overwork" of her childhood.[118] While in *Woman* she praises the pseudonymous Miranda's father for having "addressed her . . . as a living mind," her more explicitly autobiographical recollections describe the physically injurious effects of her father's expectations.[119] Fuller describes herself as an extreme case of disrupted development: "a youthful prodigy" whose rigorous intellectual education produced "premature development of the brain," which in turn "prevented the harmonious development of my bodily powers and checked my growth," leaving a pattern of "continual headache, weakness and nervous affections, of all kinds."[120] Indeed, she echoes Martineau's concerns about the physical consequences of mental "over-excitement" when she describes her own young brain as having been "in a state of being both too active and too intense, which wasted my constitution."[121] Fuller proposes that physical education could have remedied this injury, lamenting, "I do wish that I had read no books at all till later,—that I had lived with toys, and played in the open air."[122]

Scholarly attention to Fuller's youth and her account of "Miranda's" upbringing in *Woman* have presented as individual biography a dynamic that Fuller herself portrays as endemic to American education. Though she frames her youthful precocity as unusual, she insists that her miseducation was not. "No one," she declares in her "Autobiographical Romance," "understood this subject of health then."[123] Indeed, Fuller describes her father's "great mistake" as a "common" error—one she hopes will be prevented in subsequent generations by "the warnings of physiologists."[124] While she laments having had "no natural childhood," this designation marks her education as deviating not from social norms but rather from what she later called the body's "physical laws."[125] Framing her impairments as a result of systemic sexism, Fuller argues that her upbringing was similar to that of other girls in that it disregarded physiological theories of development. She draws on her understanding of her own health to advocate for broader social reform in an 1846 review of physician John C. Warren's *Physical Education and the Preservation of Health*. "Those who feel that the game of life is so nearly up with them," she advises, "should, at least, be unwilling to injure the next generation by the same ignorance which has blighted so many of us in our earliest years."[126] Her sense of her own stunted development thus led Fuller to view physical education as a vital health measure for children for whom a lifetime of able-bodiedness still remained attainable.

While critics such as Cynthia J. Davis, Deborah Manson, and Rachel A. Blumenthal have identified the significance of illness and health for Fuller's feminist transcendentalism, examining Fuller's turn to physical education also helps clarify the roles of race and nation in her conception of female health. Like many reformers, Fuller viewed cultivating individual health as inextricable from shoring up white American hegemony. She believed firmly that the bodies of white girls—and with them, the political status of white women—could be transformed by an education system that incorporated physical activity. At the same time, because she insisted that female impairment was the result of an overly sedentary life, Fuller could extend neither her critique nor her intervention to Indigenous women, whom she suggested were actually impaired by the physical demands of their social roles. Her ideas about physical education combined racial determinism with her belief that educational experiences shaped women's embodiments. Suggesting both corporeal plasticity and preexisting biological laws, Fuller espouses what Kyla Schuller has described as a prevalent nineteenth-century belief in the white body's exceptional "impressibility," or susceptibility to physiological change over time. Ultimately, Fuller's racially differentiated theories of female development both fueled her aspirations for white women's spiritual and political capacities and established the racist limitations of physical education as a tool of reform.

As Carolyn Sorisio and Susan J. Rosowski each have argued, her narration of her westward journey in *Summer on the Lakes, in 1843* reveals how the Jeffersonian ethos of American expansionism imbued in Fuller by her father seeped into her feminist and transcendentalist ideals. Fuller infuses her travel narrative with concerns about how white women's health will be established and maintained in this new extension of the nation. Both the promise of a new American frontier and the juxtaposition Fuller creates between white female physiques as harbingers of the future and Native women's bodies as remnants of the past reveal the national and racial basis of Fuller's physiological vision of reform. Indeed, Fuller describes colonial expansion itself in terms of bodily exertion when she writes that "the white settler pursues the Indian, and is victor in the chase."[127] Just as Thoreau wrote of the West, "the future lies that way to me," Fuller presents her expedition as an opportunity to reimagine white female embodiment through settler colonialist enterprise.[128]

Fuller's hope for the West echoes ideas expressed by both Wright and Martineau. Both invoked what Conevery Bolton Valenčius calls the "geography of health" by which early American settlers of the West came to view the boundary between body and environment as porous.[129] As early as 1821, Wright was particularly enthusiastic about health in the "new states."[130] If the nation as a whole is "young and vigorous," then what Wright in 1821 called the "infant West" represents an even newer locale that Wright can imbue with further potential.[131] She suggests that the "boundless territory" of the still growing United States is mirrored in the growth of its citizens.[132] "It is a singular fact," she reports, "that the citizens of the new states are often remarkable for uncommon longevity, and universally for uncommon stature," and Wright attributes this "varying standard of bodily vigor" between the eastern and western states to "less or greater pressure of mental solicitude."[133] Martineau, too, documents her travels West in *Society*. She recalls having seen in Detroit "the healthiest set of faces that I had beheld since I left England," and she deems "the State of Michigan" one of only three places where she observed "vigorous health" in the United States.[134] Fuller, however, was concerned by what she observed among a community of New Englanders who have settled in Illinois. She determines that "the great drawback upon the lives of these settlers . . . is the unfitness of the women for their new lot."[135] She recalls, "we could not but look with deep interest on the little girls and hope they would grow up with the strength of body, dexterity, simple tastes, and resources that would fit them to enjoy and refine the western farmer's life."[136] Here Fuller portrays the ideal western farmer—that personification of American expansion—as a physically strong and capable woman. The transformation of young white women into this figure, she suggests, is directly tied to the development of the nation.

Aghast at what she perceives as the "joylessness, and inaptitude, both of body and mind" of the "little girls," Fuller quickly attributes these qualities to their inadequate physical education.[137] As Cheryl J. Fish notes, Fuller saw herself in these girls and believed that "both education and rigid gender roles had contributed to her own and the prairie women's inability to adapt to their time and place."[138] Ever skeptical of the older generation's influence, Fuller holds the girls' mothers responsible, citing a disjuncture between educational models inherited from New England and their new environment. As she writes in *Woman*, "'Her mother did so before her' is no longer a sufficient excuse" for "why there should be no effort made for reformation."[139] In *Summer*, she admonishes the New England–born mothers' "mania" for a system in which pupils "learn to be quiet" and insists that the girls in Illinois need "good schools . . . planned by persons of sufficient thought to meet the wants of the place and time."[140] Fuller would later launch this same critique at all American schools for girls, proposing that the "women . . . at the head of these institutions . . . have, as yet, seldom been thinking women, capable to organize a new whole for the wants of the time."[141] Written shortly before the annexation of Texas, *Summer* takes up shifting national boundaries as an opportunity to expand women's physical education. The newness of the western locale appears to provide an urgent impetus for establishing "a kind of new, original, enchanting" model of female embodiment, one that prioritizes "bodily strength to enjoy plenty of exercise."[142] The promise of an expanded America, Fuller suggests, is also an opportunity to intervene in the embodied norms of white womanhood—and in the intellectual and spiritual capacities these might beget.

Fuller criticizes the Illinois mothers for behaving "as if the thousand needs which call out their [daughters'] young energies, and the language of nature around, yielded no education," and suggests that their daughters' physiques be developed by interacting with the new terrain they encounter.[143] The "western farmer's life" that awaits these girls will require them to not only inhabit but also actively work upon the landscape.[144] A decade before Thoreau prescribed the "tonic of wildness" in *Walden: Or, Life in the Woods* (1854) as a remedy for a host of bodily and spiritual ills, Fuller offers nature as an instructive resource and preventive measure for a new class of women whose cultivated health will facilitate their transcendence.[145] Imagining a system in which outdoor activity primes women to engage with and benefit from the landscapes they inhabit, Fuller offers an early expression of what disability studies scholar Alison Kafer describes as the ableist attachment to the rugged individualism associated with activities like hiking. This narrow approach to interacting with nature, Kafer argues, figures "able-bodiedness [as] necessary in order to bridge or transcend the essential separation between human and nature."[146] This conviction offers a key link between the influences of transcendentalist and physical education reformers on Fuller's thinking. If, for Ralph Waldo Emerson, nature is "the first in importance of the influences upon the mind," Fuller views corporeality as an essential conduit of this influence.[147] Far from "transparent eye-ball[s]," the students of whom Fuller writes are highly embodied.[148] Experiencing the "education" provided by the "language of nature," Fuller suggests, requires a "strength of body" in women unaccounted for by dominant pedagogical paradigms."[149]

The future Fuller imagines for white girls in their new western locale sharply contrasts her view of the Indigenous women she encounters in Mackinaw, Michigan, an island that Martineau described in *Society* as "so healthy" for the white settlers living there.[150] Susan Burch argues that "ableist rationales ultimately reinforce settler aspirations and further actions," and, indeed, what Jess L. Wilcox Cowing would call Fuller's "settler ableist" assessment of Native women as disabled—and inevitably so—reveals the racist limitations of her feminist physical education theories.[151] Imbuing the early American "vanishing Indian" mythology with corporeal specificity, Fuller construes the West as simultaneously a site of Native women's impairment and an impetus for white women's physical development. Fuller, Sorisio explains, "racializes herself as 'white'" by describing herself and other European American women "as corporeally and intellectually adaptable" and Native Americans as "corporeally fated."[152] Fuller describes an Indigenous "young girl, with a baby at her back" as having been "born into a world of . . . ignominious servitude and slow decay," a stark contrast to her developmental aspirations for the white daughters of Illinois farmers.[153] The edifying "language of nature" is nowhere to be seen here, but has been replaced by a contradictory environment—a "world" of "decay." These young Indigenous bodies (both of the girl and of the baby) are doomed, Fuller suggests, to a narrowly defined future of debilitating hard labor.

Fuller outlines her differential view of white and Indigenous improvability in *Woman* when she writes that, as an effect of white women's coerced dependency on men, "there is no woman, only an overgrown child," and she makes a similar though far less critical claim about "the simplicity and childish strength of the Indian race."[154] While she figures white women's disrupted development as cause for reform, she naturalizes the infantile physicality she attributes to Native people. Her observations in *Summer* reinforce this determinism. Although the manual labor that Fuller associates with Indigenous womanhood would seem to echo the "thousand needs" she claims "call out" to and develop "young energies" of the white farmer girls in Illinois, she nonetheless figures Native girls' labor as "servitude" and as the *cause* of their "decay." She confirms this trajectory in her accounts of adult Native women, whom she describes as "almost invariably coarse and ugly . . . with a peculiarly awkward gait, and forms bent by burthens" and in whom she observes "habits of drudgery expressed in their form and gesture."[155] As Sean Kicummah Teuton (Cherokee) explains, "Europeans, in perception and policy, viewed Indigenous people as . . . too defective to be repaired" and thus displaceable.[156] Indeed, Fuller suggests that Indigenous girls are subject to an entirely different developmental course than their white counterparts. While Fuller hopes the progress of American expansion represented by the "western farmer's life" will benefit the bodies of white settler girls, she simultaneously insists that the similar physical exertions or "burthens" of Native women cause their deterioration.

When she writes that Native women's "gait, so different from the steady and noble step of the men, marks the inferior position they occupy," Fuller transposes a critique of Anglo-American sexual politics onto the Indigenous women she encounters.[157] However, this portrayal of them as physically impaired by sexist society does not abide by the same logic she extends to white women's bodies. One might expect Fuller to apply her ideas about preventive health to an assimilationist position here, prefiguring the late nineteenth-century off-reservation boarding school movement's supposedly "civilizing" physical education curricula, which I discuss in chapter 4. Fuller, however, is less concerned with actual Native women than with what their experiences might represent for white female futures. As Annette Kolodny notes of *Summer*, Fuller reduces Native women to symbols of sexist oppression; her interest in them is in the service of "a further understanding of their white sisters."[158] In *Woman*, too, Fuller writes that "the Indian squaw carries the burdens of the camp" in order to refute claims that the "physical circumstances of woman would make a part in the affairs of national government unsuitable," but she makes no gestures toward Native women's participation in such political activities.[159]

More than merely exclusionary, the embodied terms of Fuller's call for reforms in physical education actually insist upon the subjugation of Native people. Her belief in the West's "limitless opportunities" for white women is mutually constituted by the irreversible deterioration she attributes to Native bodies. Throughout *Summer*, Fuller contributes to the pervasive early nineteenth-century Anglo-American conflation of natural landscapes and Native people. Despite what she describes as the "broken and degraded condition" in which she encounters them, Fuller insists that "there *was* a greatness, unique and precious" to Native people's now "defaced figures."[160]

"He who does not feel" this "greatness," Fuller claims, "will never duly appreciate the majesty of nature in this American continent."[161] She suggests that Native bodies are not only deteriorating, but in doing so also becoming materially part of the western landscape into which American borders are expanding and on which Fuller stakes her hopes for white female development.

When she quips that New England pedagogical methods "are as ill-suited to the daughter of an Illinois farmer, as satin shoes to climb the Indian mounds," she juxtaposes the impracticality of New England daintiness with the demands of a different terrain, but she also figures white female development as a triumph over a topography of which Native people are quite literally rendered part.[162] If, as Stacey Alaimo tells us, early white feminists' articulations of nature are "bound up with racist demarcations," so too is the physical strength upon which their interpolation into such natural landscapes is predicated.[163] The new feminine model that Susan Gilmore poignantly describes as "stake[d] . . . squarely on Indian (burial) ground" imagines white female bodies as improvable, and Native bodies as irrevocably ruined.[164] The image of the "Indian mounds" renders the supposedly "decay[ing]" Native women Fuller describes elsewhere in *Summer* as themselves the material foundation for white women's physical development. If Wright and Martineau emphasize the youth of the United States and its governmental structure as evidence of its potential for feminist progress, Fuller's focus on previously occupied land as a space for such edification reveals the fiction of that newness.

By asserting a model of empowered womanhood staked on physical health, Fuller leaves little room in the feminist future she imagines for bodies deemed unhealthy, including, surprisingly, those with impairments such as she herself experienced. She justifies her own disqualification from this ideal by attributing her impairment to a sedentary youth indoors: "it is too late" for her. In contrast, her portrayal of Native women as "bent" by their physical labors offers a more essentialist explanation for their displacement from both the nation and her feminist politics. Indeed, according to Fuller, young Native girls are doomed to "decay" despite their outdoor exertions. These girls, Fuller suggests, are innately ineligible—perhaps even unfit—for a physical education agenda that promises to improve women's bodies and social roles, leaving no place for Indigenous women in the political landscape Fuller imagines.[165] By attaching political potential to the cultivation of white female bodies, Fuller's physical education advocacy is both potentially enabling for some and ultimately inextricable from the shoring up of white hegemony within the American landscape. While Fuller deemed the bodies of

Native women as outside the purview of physical education, the question of whether and how to attend to such racialized women's bodies became a crucial concern for subsequent physical education advocates. As I demonstrate in subsequent chapters, diverse forms of physical education were varyingly taken up and critiqued by later nineteenth-century feminists as mechanisms for forging just the kind of national identity Fuller hoped able-bodied white women would assume.

CHAPTER TWO

Household Health in the Domestic's Novel

While Fuller cast racialized women and girls whom she deemed inferior as ineligible for physical education, one of her earliest influences took a slightly different approach. In her domestic manual, *The Young Lady's Friend* (1838), Fuller's adolescent friend and mentor Eliza Ware Farrar not only provides her young middle-class readers with physical education advice; she also positions them as potential instructors in their own right.[1] In a chapter entitled "Treatment of Domestics and Work-Women," Farrar encourages her readers to share their health knowledge with the women and girls employed in their family homes:

> You can also enlighten them on the subject of their health, and teach them how they can best obviate the evils incident to their way of life. You can exhort them to take exercise in the open air, and show them the danger of not doing so. You can tell them the mischiefs which arise from not being sufficiently clothed, and from eating cake, sweetmeats, and pastry, between meals. If you have made yourself acquainted with the best means of preserving health, you will be able to lecture well on this important subject, and may do a great deal of good to a class of females, whose lives are now rendered burdensome by disease, or prematurely cut short by death.[2]

For Farrar, "domestics," or household laborers, constitute a *"class* of females" in two senses; these laborers are defined as a distinct population by their socioeconomic standing, and they also represent pupils whom her readers are positioned to instruct. Tenets of physical education such as proper exercise, clothing, and diet are given here as evidence of middle- and upper-class "young ladies'" moral superiority—their knowledge of these subjects equips them to eradicate "evil" habits in the domestic workers laboring in their homes. In reality, though, domestics were largely responsible for providing for many of Farrar's readers' own health through the performance of household chores. Any disproportionate tendencies to "disease" and "premature[] . . . death" they themselves displayed were likely the result not of inadequate health knowledge but of overwork.[3]

That Farrar positions physical education, rather than labor reform, as a solution to this health crisis shows how the rhetoric of physical education could be used to belie the power dynamics inherent in the employer/domestic relationship. While chapter 1 focused primarily on outdoor exercise as a means through which women's health expertise made its way across the expanding terrain of the United States, this chapter centers on the home as a locus of physical education practices including hygienic and culinary labor. Such chores, which were framed as necessary to promoting the health of the household, were not only performed but also taught. Much as Fuller deemed the mothers she met in Illinois responsible for providing the next generation with a physical education suited to their western environment, middle-class New England women assigned themselves the task of providing instruction in proper American domestic labor practices not only to their own daughters but also to the women they employed. In the nineteenth century, the domestic/employer relationship was coded in expressly pedagogical terms. Indeed, even as they required them to perform domestic labor, many middle-class women imagined domestics as pupils incapable of managing a healthy home without their oversight.

Though the pedagogical dynamic between middle-class women and their often quite young employees sometimes mirrored their training of these women's own daughters, the racialization of domestic labor produced a particularly vexed maternalistic model of physical education. Building on scholarship on childhood as both experience and ideology in the nineteenth-century United States, this chapter examines narratives about actual child laborers as well as rhetorical constructions of racialized domestics as perpetually childlike and therefore in need of instruction.[4] As a form of care that sociologist Evelyn Nagano Glenn refers to as the "racialized gendered servitude" born of legal apparatuses and social inequities, nineteenth-century domestic work positioned laborers as at once caregivers and dependents.[5] Domestic service was the most common occupation for working women in the nineteenth-century United States, and the majority of these were Irish immigrants and Black women.[6] Many young women entered into service seeking access to the privileges associated with middle-class whiteness — including both the financial gain of employment and the health knowledge that would equip them to oversee their own future homes and families. As Amy Kaplan has famously argued, the discourse of domesticity was an instrument of empire, and the threshold of the home came to stand in for the nation's shifting borders.[7] The presence of a "foreign" child or supposedly childlike presence in the home thus coded that space as an arena in which middle-class white women could exert political power through physical education instruction.

Exertions of this power and the resultant (mis)education of workers are on full display in domestic novels that critique the cultures of abuse and neglect that pervaded domestic service arrangements. The genre of "domestic fiction," which focused on young heroines overcoming adversity in their home lives, provided mid-nineteenth-century women with a framework for exploring the tumultuous social relationships that played out within the home. Rather than demarcate women's concerns to a limited sphere, the genre positioned female influence as expansive by imagining "everyone was to be placed in the home, and hence home and the world would become one."[8] This chapter turns to two writers who drew on tropes of domestic fiction in order to interrogate the nature of domestic service: Catharine Maria Sedgwick and Harriet Wilson. In their contributions to a subgenre we might call "the domestic's novel," these writers illustrate both the expectations of physical education and maternal guidance that domestics brought with them to service and the ways in which employers could abuse their authority to cause domestics physical injury. Sedgwick's and Wilson's novels make these volatile pedagogical relationships visible, and they also provide instructive insight for readers by illustrating how prevailing service models harm racialized domestics.

In this chapter, I begin by establishing the maternalist view of domestic service codified in the advice manuals of Catharine Beecher, for whom physical education and household labor were closely intertwined. Addressing employers and employees alike in separate manuals directed at each audience, Beecher delineates the pedagogical function of service and the racial limitations for receiving that tutelage. From there, I turn to Sedgwick's and Wilson's domestic's novels, which I argue illustrate both the possibilities and failures of framing service as physical education through extended depictions of employers' (mis)education of domestics.

Catharine Beecher and the "Care" of Domestics

Perhaps no one was more adamant in characterizing domestics as students of physical education than Catharine Beecher, the older sister of abolitionist novel *Uncle Tom's Cabin; or, Life among the Lowly* (1852) author Harriet Beecher Stowe. After founding the Hartford Female Seminary in Hartford, Connecticut, in 1823 and teaching there for nearly a decade, Beecher extended the reach of her pedagogy by publishing her instruction in a slew of domestic advice books for women and young girls. In the most famous of these, the widely read *A Treatise on Domestic Economy: For the Use of Young Ladies at Home, and at School* (1841), Beecher calls on her young, white, middle-class readers to adopt a maternal attitude toward the domestics she imagines they will someday employ. In a chapter titled "On the Care of Domestics," she echoes Farrar in making the case that though they may be responsible for the physical comforts of their employers, domestics in fact need guidance in matters of health. Beecher addresses the much-bemoaned frequency with which domestics apparently leave their posts, and she attributes this high turnover rate to employers' mismanagement. In order to retain their employees, she recommends that housewives "attach domestics to the family."[9] Doing so, according to Beecher, not only requires the provision of material comforts such as "comfortable rooms, and good food" but also involves "guarding [domestics'] health," in part by teaching them "how to improve."[10] Employers, she explains, must "supply the place of parents," since "the management of both domestics and of children" requires similar methods of patience and gentle instruction in order to "cure defects" in both.[11] By "attach[ing]" them to the families they served in this way, Beecher advocates for treating domestics, regardless of their age, as childlike pupils.

Beecher offered the kind of instruction she championed in a new publication the following year.[12] In *Letters to Persons Who Are Engaged in Domestic Service* (1842), Beecher addresses domestics directly, instructing them, among other things, to "take good care of your health."[13] In a strikingly threatening section, Beecher warns her readers of the particular risks of their falling ill as compared to persons who have "wealth and a comfortable home" such as their employers.[14] "When you are sick," she declares, "you have no parents or family friends around you, to nurse and sympathize; you know that the family you live in have not only lost your services, but are obliged to wait upon you, and you feel that you are a burden."[15] Beecher not only makes the bold assumption that domestics are entirely lacking in community outside their place of employment; she also delineates limitations on their childlike status within the families with whom they live. It is not so much that domestics have no one to care for their physical body should they become sick, but rather that their need for care when ill disrupts the economic relationship in which employers benefit from rather than provide "services." She warns them to avoid becoming a "burden" and an object of charity, rather than a member of the "honourable and respectable class" of domestics who provide for "the comfort, health, and prosperity" of a "society" of which they clearly are not considered part.[16]

To prevent such a disruption to the domestic status quo and maintain their respectability, Beecher implores her readers to heed the health advice printed in both her *Letters* and her *Treatise*. "Much of the ill health among persons in your employment," she insists in the chapter "On Health," "is entirely needless."[17] She laments the frequency with which domestics across the country are "wearing down their constitutions, without being aware of it" before proceeding to list a series of unhealthy habits that she fails to acknowledge generally fall beyond the purview of domestics' control.[18] She reports their propensity for overworking, wearing inadequate clothing, and sleeping in poorly ventilated rooms—all of which are the responsibility of their employers—and suggests that these are the result of their own ignorance.

As evidence that any illness is due to their failure to care for themselves properly, Beecher suggests that domestics are in fact occupationally predisposed to health, since they engage in "employments . . . that tend to strengthen the constitution and maintain firm health."[19] Beecher describes domestic labor similarly in her *Treatise* in the chapter "On Domestic Exercise." In that section, Beecher displays the belief in the benefits of domestic labor that Harriet Martineau critiqued by arguing that proper performance of household chores was conducive to young women's physical and mental health. Beecher also encourages readers of *Letters* to consult the chapter "On the Care of Health" in her *Treatise* in order to develop a fuller understanding of their anatomy that she promises will equip them to perform their labor healthfully. Domestic service, she ultimately implies, could be a form of physical education for otherwise ignorant, working-class women seeking "a state of constant training" in household labor under the careful supervision of their more knowledgeable middle-class employers.[20] In fact, Beecher cautions readers that leaving domestic service in pursuit of other professions could put their health at risk. "I have known cases," she reports, "where young girls have left the place of a domestic in a good family, to go to shops or manufactories, who, after the trial, have returned with broken down health."[21] This claim, which runs counter to historian Faye Dudden's finding that physical exhaustion drove many domestics to leave their posts, shows that the promise of health was a tactic used to frame domestic service as an edifying occupation.[22]

Beecher's threat clearly results from her sense of domestic labor as an industry in crisis. "I hope," she writes in the introduction to her *Letters*, "to make you more useful, and more contented with your lot," suggesting that her concern for their health stems from a desire to keep them in service.[23] In her *Treatise*, Beecher confesses to her middle-class readers that the American context begets particular challenges for retaining domestics. She explains that unlike in the aristocratic European nations upon which American service is modeled, the possibility of class ascension in the United States means that the number of households able to afford live-in service is ever increasing, and the number of young women in economic need, and thus willing to enter the profession, is declining.[24] The lack of domestics, she reports, has increased the burdens on middle-class housewives, leaving them "disheartened, discouraged, and ruined in health."[25]

The racial and national anxieties that undergird Beecher's equation of domestics with children surface in her description of this crisis. As Andrew Urban has shown, the reluctance of white, US-born workers to enter service was a product of the increasing racialization of such labor, a shift that Beecher feared would have immense consequences.[26] While the Irish and Black women workers who dominated the field of domestic service were certainly characterized as childlike and ignorant, writers like Beecher denied the possibility that they could receive the same training as white, US-born domestics and, with it, the same care.[27] Beecher's *Treatise* juxtaposes the "well-trained domestics" whom she would later address in her *Letters* with the "ignorant foreigners" and "shiftless slaves" on whom middle-class American women must rely in the absence of US-born white labor.[28] She provides the example of a former student of hers who, upon marrying and having a child, found that "*her health failed*; while, for most of the time, she had no domestics, at all, or only Irish or Germans, who scarcely knew even the names, or the uses of many cooking utensils."[29] The retention of US-born white women in domestic service, according to Beecher, is a boon not only to their health but also to that of those who employ them. While she suggested that domestic skills can be taught through a process of physical education, she also insisted that aptitude for learning was racially determined. In her *Treatise*, she explains that American women have "inherited" their housekeeping "tastes and habits" from their "English progenitors, who, as a nation, are distinguished for systematic housekeeping, and for a great love of order, cleanliness, and comfort."[30] According to Beecher's logic, the ideal, trainable domestic was akin to her employer's daughter and thus must share her racial lineage.

As such, Beecher's vision of an ideal domestic service industry harkens back to an earlier American arrangement known as "help." Over the course of the nineteenth century, US homes gradually transitioned away from this model in which young women assisted neighbors with domestic chores as part of an interpersonal and temporary relationship rather than a professional commitment of long-term service. As a common developmental stage in a young woman's life rather than a subordinate and possibly permanent status, "help" lacked the class and race associations of wage-earning domestic service. Dudden has shown that as the nature of outsourced household labor shifted over the course of the century, the labels of "help" and "domestic" functioned more as "models or ideal types" than fixed designations, and tracing the way the two categories map onto race provides a useful framework for interpreting disparities in the treatment of domestic workers.

While the maternalism espoused by Beecher and others positioned domestics, regardless of age, as childlike, ideas about race shaped the developmental trajectory employers imagined for them. The idea of childhood was itself a racially demarcated designation, and this extended to the view of domestics as either capable of growth or occupying a permanent state of dependence. Retaining the familial bonds established by the "help" model of labor, Anglo-American domestics could be understood as surrogate daughters in need of a physical education that would prepare them to oversee their own future households. Immigrant and Black workers, on the other hand, were often framed both as ignorant juveniles in need of supervision and as fundamentally incapable of meaningful improvement. As such, the physical education that domestic service provided was not an equalizing tool that facilitated widespread class mobility, but was rather differentially applied based on racial categories.

Health Knowledge and Class Mobility in *Live and Let Live*

When Beecher reminds *Treatise*'s readers of their responsibility to provide for their domestics, she supplements this guidance with a footnote directing them to a fictional text. She writes, "The excellent little work of Miss Sedgwick, entitled 'Live, and Let Live,' contains many valuable and useful hints, conveyed in a most pleasing narrative form, which every housekeeper would do well to read."[31] Published in 1837, *Live and Let Live; or, Domestic Service Illustrated* was one of three didactic novels Sedgwick published after the Reverend Henry Ware urged her to pen "a series of narratives, between a formal tale and a common tract" that would illustrate the value of Christian morality.[32] Indeed, the narrator of *Live and Let Live* oscillates between tropes of sentimentality and the instructive tone of domestic manuals. The novel tells the story of thirteen-year-old Lucy Lee, whose previously prosperous family has fallen into poverty as a result of her father's alcoholism. After her mother resolves to find her daughter employment as a domestic, Lucy undertakes a host of short-term positions in different women's homes. As the novel follows Lucy from one workplace to another, it models the ideal employer or "mistress" by highlighting the virtues of some characters and the harmful attitudes of others.[33] Through periodic commentary assessing the behavior of the various women for whom Lucy works, the didactic novel that Sedgwick hoped would do "some little good to the high and the humble" exposes middle-class women's dangerous disregard for their domestics' well-being and models an alternative approach grounded in health knowledge.[34] Notably, she does not suggest that household labor revert to a precapitalist model of "help," but rather that the relationship between domestics and their employers be transformed to make service more tenable.[35] When read in the context of the physical education domestics expected to receive from the women who employed them, the "family-like affect" that Barbara Ryan rightly identifies as central to *Live and Let Live*'s vision emerges as a call not only for moral reform but for health reform as well.[36]

As Beecher would later suggest, the ideal employer for Sedgwick is akin to a mother who possesses thorough knowledge of what the narrator of *Live and Let Live* describes as "that science which every woman should study, domestic economy" and draws on that expertise "to raise the character of domestic laborers."[37] Despite Lucy's family's evident economic necessity (the novel's opening scene shows them unable to afford a loaf of bread, and the family of six sleeps in a single room), the text presents her domestic service not only as a source of much needed income, but also as an opportunity for her to receive a physical education. Indeed, upon commencing her work, the narrator reports that "Lucy, while serving others, was educating herself."[38] As they seek a position for Lucy, the Lees encounter a host of potential employers, whose failings are made evident by their reluctance to employ young girls who "require[] too much teaching" or, as one puts it, to "turn a gentleman's house into school!"[39] Lucy's development, however, is at the forefront of Mrs. Lee's mind as she searches for "a good place, where the weaknesses of childhood would be considered; where its faults would be patiently borne with, forgiven, and corrected; where its ignorance would be instructed; and where the employer would feel the responsibility, and the privilege, we may add, of training a young creature."[40] Toward the novel's end, Lucy finally finds such a place in the home of Mrs. Hyde, who specifically prefers "young subjects" as her domestics because they "can be remoulded and taught," and, indeed, Lucy finds herself "daily acquiring knowledge in the domestic arts" under her supervision.[41]

Throughout the novel, health knowledge is central to the narrator's assessment of Lucy's various employers' aptitudes for the role of mistress. On her first day at Mrs. Broadson's, for instance, Lucy quickly learns a handful of health maxims, including that tea and coffee are "unhealthy," that "it's bad to be idle," and that "it's a bad habit to keep running to the fire" for warmth."[42] Another employer, Mrs. Ardley, is portrayed as ignorant of "the first principles of physiology," having "not yet learned that it was her duty to know the actual conditions of her domestics, to watch over their health."[43] As a result, Lucy is overworked and exposed to significant cold, which causes her to develop inflammation of the lungs. When Lucy takes to her bed in the unheated servants' quarters, Mrs. Ardley is certain this will not impede her healing, since "servants are accustomed to cold rooms."[44] Notably, it is her young daughter, Anne, who points out that domestics, like the Ardleys themselves, also spend "part of their time in . . . warm rooms" and thus might appreciate the comfort.[45] This recognition of domestics' physiological needs prompts an overhearing servant to remark of Anne that "the child is fit to be a mistress," and the narrator notes that "difficulties" such as Lucy's illness "would be materially lessened if young women were educated for their household duties."[46]

The young Anne Ardley embodies the novel's implicit claim that preparation for overseeing domestics is an essential element of middle-class girlhood.[47] "It is indispensable," Mrs. Hyde remarks at one point, "to give our daughters a thorough acquaintance with domestic affairs."[48] Here Mrs. Hyde expresses one of the novel's central theses—and Sedgwick's own attitude. It is "imperative," Sedgwick insists in the novel's preface, for "American mothers to qualify their daughters to superintend their domestics."[49] Later on, the narrator looks ahead optimistically to a time "when physical, intellectual, and moral education will have raised the level of our race, and brought it to as near an approximation to equality of condition as it is capable of in its present state of existence."[50] Training future mistresses for their adult responsibilities, the novel proposes, will elevate the health and character of the women who serve them.

At the same time, the novel suggests that instilling middle-class ideals in domestics themselves will enable their socioeconomic mobility. Both Lucy's mother and her eventual ideal employer, Mrs. Hyde, view Lucy's domestic employment as preparation for middle-class womanhood. Early on in the novel, Mrs. Lee assures her dubious husband that "in a well-ordered family, a [domestic] is fitting herself for the duties that belong to her sex. She is learning to fill honorably the station of a wife, mistress, and mother of a family."[51] Committed to this ideal, she even turns down a home where her daughter would be tasked with minimal work because she believes Lucy "must be qualifying herself for the future" and "the very light work she has here would rather unfit than fit her for the future."[52] That prospective employer stands in stark contrast to Mrs. Hyde, who is able "to qualify those she employed for the happier condition that probably awaited them—to be the masters and mistresses of independent homes."[53] This dynamic positions Lucy as a parallel to Mrs. Hyde's own daughter, Susan, whom Lucy is surprised to see sharing in her household labor. Lucy is stunned to learn that in this house "young ladies rise as early as the servants," and further shocked by Mrs. Hyde's "acknowledgement that all the members were governed by the same physical laws."[54] The conflation of the roles of domestic and daughter are made explicit at the novel's conclusion when Lucy reports to Mrs. Lee, "In all respects Mrs. Hyde has been a mother to me. She has qualified me to take charge of a family of my own."[55]

By suggesting that Lucy will eventually become a "mistress" of her own home, the novel grants her a degree of socioeconomic mobility that, as it makes plain elsewhere, was reserved for only those Anglo-American women whose presence in the home carried the connotations of familial "help." The extent to which race enables Lucy to occupy this daughter-like status comes into focus when she enters service at Mrs. Broadson's home. There, she meets Bridget (called "Biddy" by the other characters), who is introduced in the text as "an Irish servant" and who, during Lucy's interview with Mrs. Broadson, "kindly drew a chair for Lucy to the fire."[56] Her first line of dialogue, "warm ye, child," differentiates her from Lucy through both the use of dialect and her apparent maturity in comparison to this "child" whose ill health she observes and works to ameliorate.[57] However, the narrator's gloss of this gesture reduces Bridget's maternal concern for Lucy's physical well-being to a mere "kind word," foreshadowing the novel's later differentiation between Bridget's apparently strictly emotional approach to care and Lucy's more informed domestic scientific knowledge.[58]

Indeed, when overseen by Bridget, the fire's warmth becomes less a health tonic than a metaphor for certain personality traits; Sedgwick saw the Irish as possessing an "element of *warmth* and generosity" that she hoped they would "infus[e]" into the American "national character."[59] Sedgwick's view of Irish women as governed by feeling is evident in the novel's portrayal of Bridget as an overly emotional and thus ineffective caregiver. Shortly after her introduction, readers learn that Bridget maintains a close relationship with her niece, Judy M'Phealan, who Bridget hopes Mrs. Broadson will someday employ.[60] When Judy falls ill, Bridget's response is portrayed as largely emotional. After hearing of her niece's manifold symptoms, she "burst[s] into tears" and later laments, "what in the world am I to do with her?"[61] This apparent inability to respond rationally to Judy's illness aligns Bridget with a trope already implied by her nickname. Throughout the mid-nineteenth century, women's magazines printed fictional stories about the "Irish Biddy," a stock character defined by coarseness and ineptitude.[62] Sedgwick herself adopted this view of Irish domestics. Although she wrote in 1853 that she was "grateful for Irish servants" as a needed alternative to what she saw as "shiftless, lazy, and unfaithful" Black women workers, Sedgwick also viewed the Irish as plagued by "their Celtic infirmities on their heads—their half savage ways—their blunders—their imaginativeness—indefiniteness—and curve-lines every way."[63] By characterizing these women as both "infirm" and "half savage," Sedgwick simultaneously medicalizes and racializes them in order to explain their alleged incompetence. Crafting a racial spectrum of caregiving abilities, she positions the Irish as superior to their Black counterparts but also as less fully developed than US-born workers such as Lucy.

It is unsurprising, then, that it is Lucy who ultimately devises a plan for Judy's care in *Live and Let Live*. Throughout the girl's illness, Lucy is framed as a far more knowledgeable and effective caregiver than Bridget. If, as the text claims, "domestic economy is a science that brings into action the qualities of the mind as well as the graces of the heart," then the overly sentimental Irish are only partly fit to carry out these tasks.[64] Indeed, the narrator reports that while Bridget weeps for her ailing niece, Lucy is "more in the habit of remedying an evil than crying over it."[65] Upon the onset of Judy's illness, "Lucy was the first to observe and remark that she did not look well."[66] From here on, Lucy displays the "highest mental endowments" that the narrator elsewhere claims are essential to "the best housekeeper."[67] When Judy wakes with a cough in the night, Bridget implores Lucy to summon a priest, believing that death is near. Lucy on the other hand, not only deems the condition curable but has already prepared a warm bath that she believes will soothe the suffering girl. Her confident approach is soon validated by a physician whose "prescriptions harmoniz[e] with the restoratives Lucy had advised," and Judy recovers shortly thereafter.[68]

Lucy, the novel makes clear, is uniquely prepared to manage the health of others. Bridget is stunned by the extent of Lucy's domestic scientific knowledge, asking, "how should ye know everything, and ye such a childer?"[69] The protagonist responds by describing her own family: "it's having our Jemmie always sick, and mother to teach me."[70] Lucy's advantage, the novel makes clear, derives having observed her own "mother's way" of treating illnesses.[71] The notion that Anglo-American women provided the best instruction in domestic science bolstered both the widespread preference for US-born domestics and the perception of immigrant workers of all ages as children in need of tutelage. Sedgwick's novel endorses this view: Lucy's access to valuable maternal wisdom is presented as an explicitly Anglo-American advantage when Bridget laments, "poor Judy! All her mother did for her was to bring her into this miserable world."[72]

The novel goes on to describe standard Irish upbringing as the antithesis of the training Lucy apparently received in her American home despite her poverty: "They have bred in miserable dirty cabins, where they had *no* means of learning the arts of domestic economy."[73] The narrator explains the importance of countering such upbringing through proper training: "The Irish come to us with their habits formed. . . . Some of them may be unteachable and irreclaimable; but, for the most part, do they not repay *real* disinterested kindness with fidelity and affection? It is very common to say, 'There is no use in trying to teach an Irish person.' Is an Irish person less docile than any other who has arrived to maturity in ignorance?"[74] Here Irish women occupy a hybrid position as simultaneously "formed" and mature as well as defined by their "ignorance." They are presented as both unteachable and in urgent need of instruction. The novel's ideal of the American middle-class woman, Mrs. Hyde, expresses a similar sentiment when she bemoans "foreigners" who "have minds so stinted, and such inveterate bad habits that it is very difficult to make them comfortable members of a little family community."[75] Bridget's employer, Mrs. Broadson, too, endorses this perception. She deems Bridget an exception to the rule that Irish women are "sluttish" "and difficult to teach."[76] Bridget, in Mrs. Broadson's assessment, is "a woman of great strength, capacity, and industry . . . she accomplished more work than two ordinary women; and that all her work was well done."[77] This belief in Bridget's exceptional abilities, however, is undermined later in the narrative when Bridget tells Lucy about an earlier employer who educated her in just the fashion Mrs. Lee deemed essential for Lucy's own training. "Everything I know I learned there," Bridget declares of her time working for Mrs. Tilson, who she recalls "showed me the right way to do this, and tached [sic] me the right way to do t'other."[78] By belatedly revealing this backstory to the reader, Sedgwick counters claims that Irish women cannot be taught at all, signaling instead the importance of providing such women workers with proper training.

Sedgwick frames such supervision as an explicitly imperial project. In the novel's preface, she expresses her hope to "incite even a few of my young countrywomen to a zealous devotion to '*home missions*.'"[79] Mirroring her description elsewhere of Irish women as "half savage," she portrays domestic instruction as a civilizing endeavor. She similarly claimed in 1853 that, in the United States, the Irish "till and are tilled," suggesting that they are at once laborers and, much like the bodies beneath the "Indian mounds" Fuller described in *Summer on the Lakes*, the material environment upon which Anglo-Americans might work.[80] In *Live and Let Live*, it is not her employer, Mrs. Broadson, but Lucy herself who "tills" Bridget into performing domestic health labor properly. The narrator explains that Irish women "require knowledge, energy, and patience on the part of their employers," and Lucy herself demonstrates these qualities when educating Bridget.[81] Despite her youth, Lucy's racial status positions her as Bridget's superior and allows her to transition seamlessly from a domestic in need of education into a mistress-in-training. In overseeing and managing the incompetent Bridget, she aligns herself with the ideals of middle-class domesticity, fitting her to eventually run a home of her own.

Frado's "New Discipline"

While the white, US-born Lucy Lee of *Live and Let Live* fulfills the promise of her domestic training by becoming mistress of her own home, such a fate eludes Frado, the protagonist of Harriet Wilson's *Our Nig; or, Sketches from the Life of a Free Black in a Two-Story White House, North* (1859). Though published more than twenty years after Sedgwick's text, Wilson's autobiographical novel is seemingly set during the 1830s and '40s, when Wilson herself worked as an indentured servant for the Hayward family of Milford, New Hampshire.[82] Born in that state to a Black father and a white mother, Wilson's pseudonymous protagonist, six-year-old Frado, is left by her mother and stepfather at the home of the Bellmonts (stand-ins for the Haywards, a local family), where she works without pay until she turns eighteen. Throughout the novel, the racialization of innocence as white forecloses the possibility of both the care and the physical education that might secure young Frado's future.[83] During her long years with the Bellmonts, Frado suffers from overwork and brutal beatings that don't just replace edifying health instruction but actually cause chronic impairment. Drawing together tropes of sentimentality, seduction, gothic novels, and narratives of enslavement, Wilson's novel consistently suggests that the care Frado is denied causes her ill health and persistent pain.[84] Indeed, Wilson introduces herself to her readers in the preface as both "deserted by kindred, disabled by failing health," positioning the two side by side to illuminate their correlation.[85] If Sedgwick suggests that a domestic worker's acquisition of health knowledge from maternal figures can facilitate her economic mobility, Wilson shows how the denial of such motherly instruction for racialized workers can leave them severely debilitated and consequently destitute.[86]

Scholars have long recognized motherhood as a central value on which Wilson's narrative turns: Frado is betrayed by both her birth mother and the surrogate mother she seeks during her servitude, and the text's framing makes clear that providing for her own child's well-being was a core motivation for Wilson's writing.[87] Of all the novel's maternal figures, Frado's abusive "mistress," Mrs. Bellmont, receives the most extended depiction, placing the novel in close conversation with treatises such as Beecher's on the pedagogical expectations attached to the domestic/employer relationship. While the maternalism toward Irish adult workers illustrated in *Live and Let Live* shows how the idea of childhood could be used to marginalize immigrant women's knowledge, here an actual child worker's racialization bars her from receiving the maternal instruction imposed on adult immigrant women. The "dependence and care" that, as Karen Sánchez-Eppler argues, Wilson insists on the importance of represent a combination of the child worker's emotional, economic, and physiological needs that are neglected by exploitative employers.[88]

Following Gretchen Short, I read Wilson's portrayal of a domestic laborer as a window onto how the unstable classifications of foreign and national are played out through contested authority over the home.[89] This inquiry into the nature of domestic belonging begins in the novel's first chapters, which open not with Frado's labor, but with that of her mother, Mag Smith. Though not a live-in "domestic" per se, Mag earns her living by performing the demanding task of laundry or "washing" for middle-class families including the Bellmonts.[90] Mag, we learn, was "early deprived of parental guardianship, far removed from relatives, she was left to guide her tiny boat over life's surges alone and inexperienced."[91] Wilson's nautical metaphor doesn't just foreshadow Frado's later lack of guidance, but also alludes to the experiences of European immigrant women who traveled by boat to the United States alone at a young age in search of domestic employment. This allusion to immigrant women echoes Mag's racialization elsewhere in the text.[92] Her name, Mag Smith, implies Irish heritage, and the novel's exclusive use of the nickname "Mag" rather than the more formal "Margaret" recalls the derogatory use of "Biddy" as a shorthand not only for "Bridget" but also for all Irish domestics.[93]

As such, the novel marks Mag as belonging to the derided class of outsider domestics that her daughter will shortly join.

Furthermore, although her eventual husband and Frado's father, Jim, identifies her as his "white wife," he also recognizes that she occupies a unique status within the racial classification system of the Northeast. Having been ostracized by the white community after bearing a child out of wedlock, Mag, Jim muses, would "be as much of a prize to me as she'd fall short of coming up to the mark with white folks."[94] Indeed, reporting on a week of labor, she tells Jim, "I washed for the Reeds, and did a small job for Mrs. Bellmont; that's all. I shall starve soon, unless I can get more to do. Folks seem as afraid to come here as if they expected to get some awful disease."[95] Wilson frames Mag's alienation from these women by invoking racialized claims about working women's health. By equating her stigmatization to an unhygienic home, the novel recalls Sedgwick's discussion of Irish immigrant women in *Live and Let Live* as having been "bred in miserable dirty cabins, where they had *no* means of learning the arts of domestic economy."[96] Foretelling Frado's experience later in the novel, Mag is not only alienated from her family of origin but also unable to find a substitute for such absent maternal guidance among the women who employ her.[97]

When Mag abandons Frado at the Bellmont house, claiming that she will return after completing a washing job for a neighboring family, she reproduces her own "remov[al]" from relatives by removing her daughter from her own home. The parallel orphaning of mother and daughter is further underscored in a letter by "Margaret Thorn" that was published in the novel's appendix.[98] There, Thorn writes of the protagonist, "being taken from home so young, and placed where she had nothing to love or cling to, I often wonder she had not grown up a *monster*."[99] This account invokes the earlier characterization of Mag's failings as a result of her lack of familial guidance, and it also challenges that logic. Frado, in contrast, is portrayed as fully human despite her mother's neglect. This act of maternal disavowal does, however, have a significant impact on Frado's story.[100] When Frado tells a member of the Bellmont family, "I ha'n't got no mother, no home. I wish I was dead," she reveals the depths of her despair, and she foretells the ensuing destruction of her physical body that the novel suggests better mothering might have prevented.[101]

Mag is not the only woman who fails to care for Frado. Though no formal agreement between Mag and Mrs. Bellmont is described in the text, the narrator reports that a year after her abandonment, Frado was deemed

Household Health in the Domestic's Novel 51

"a permanent member of the family," and this surrogate family, too, leaves Frado without maternal oversight.[102] Importantly, the "Thorn" letter doesn't just criticize Mag's abandonment of her child, it also notes that young Frado was "placed where she had nothing to love or cling to."[103] Much as Sedgwick demonstrates the failings of many of the women who employ domestic workers, Wilson makes plain that Mrs. Bellmont is ill-suited for her role. Mag acknowledges this when she admits that as a result of Mrs. Bellmont's "ugly" qualities, "she can't keep a girl in the house over a week."[104] Mrs. Bellmont herself attributes these frequent turnovers to the age of her usual "girls." "I have so much trouble with girls I hire," she tells her daughter, Mary, "I am almost persuaded if I have one to train up in my way from a child, I shall be able to keep them awhile. I am tired of changing every few months."[105] As the novel progresses, however, her brand of "train[ing]" disrupts rather than aids Frado's development and ultimately proves dangerous to her young charge.

Referring to her household responsibilities as "a new discipline to the child," Wilson both alludes to the possibility that Frado might receive proper physical education at the Bellmonts' and foreshadows the injurious treatment that she receives instead.[106] On the rare occasion when Mrs. Bellmont does instruct Frado in proper methods of completing her chores, such as "how [feeding the hens] was *always* to be done," she undermines these moments of instruction with physical abuse—"departure from this rule [was] . . . punished by a whipping."[107] Her supervision of Frado is both ineffective and violent: "It was her favorite exercise to enter the apartment noisily, vociferate orders, give a few sudden blows to quicken [Frado's] pace, then return to the sitting room with *such* a satisfied expression, congratulating herself upon her thorough house-keeping qualities."[108] By ironically characterizing Mrs. Bellmont's verbal and physical abuse as "house-keeping," the novel underscores the extent to which Frado's status within the Bellmont home perverts the pedagogical relationship on which domestic service was premised and, in doing so, exposes its racist underpinnings.

The depth of Mrs. Bellmont's failings as a housekeeper are further illuminated when she leaves town and Mary is "installed housekeeper—in name merely, for [Frado] was the only moving power in the house."[109] As the novel's subtitle suggests, the Bellmont residence is indeed a "two-story" home, and this scene in which "name" and actual "power" diverge reveals the discrepancy between those two disparate domestic narratives.[110] Given that writers like Beecher and Sedgwick viewed proper supervision of domestics as an important aspect of middle-class white women's training, Mary's treatment of Frado can be read as an illustration of her mother's approach to education. As temporary "housekeeper," Mary not only fails to perform any chores herself; she also provides inaccurate instruction, "insist[ing] upon some compliance to her wishes in some department which she was very imperfectly acquainted with, very much less than the person she was addressing."[111] The incompetence Mary has apparently inherited from her mother makes clear that any skills Frado has acquired have been procured through experience and not as a result of Mrs. Bellmont's maternal supervision. Mary, we learn, has also inherited her mother's use of physical abuse as a means of supervising household chores. When Frado falls ill and fails to promptly answer Mary's call for her to sweep, Mary throws "a large carving knife" at her.[112] As the weaponized kitchen tool makes clear, Mrs. Bellmont's domestic instruction puts domestic's bodies in danger. Indeed, Mrs. Bellmont "did not trouble herself about the future destiny of her servant. If she did what she desired for *her* benefit, it was all the responsibility she acknowledged."[113] Though this line appears in a section about Frado's religious education and possible salvation, the later economic impacts of her injuries by Mrs. Bellmont make clear that Frado's more immediate, earthly future was equally immaterial to her. Frado, in her eyes, is an instrument of her own well-being rather than a child for whom she is responsible.

Frado, who begins her service at age six, is in fact a child, though she is rarely treated as such. The novel frames her twelve-year tenure at the Bellmonts' as a formative period in Frado's development and an era which should occasion some maternal instruction. Recalling the contracts of white "bound girls" who traded their domestic services to wealthier families in exchange for residential and educational advantages, Frado eventually resolves not to run away but "to stay contentedly through her period of service, which would expire when she was eighteen years of age."[114] While Frado's age and orphaning liken her plight to that of actual bound girls in New Hampshire during the 1830s, she receives none of the healthful training that such arrangements promised to provide.[115] Though bonding was intended as an "almost adoptive relationship," Frado's responsibilities in the Belmont home are far from those of a daughter.[116] Her domestic chores, we're routinely told, are inappropriate for and potentially damaging to her young frame, causing a state of chronic physical and psychological stress that Crystal S. Donkor notes would now be recognized as an elevated "allostatic load" predictive of poor health in the future.[117] Within a year of her service, "she was quite indispensable, although but seven years old," completing outsized tasks such as "a large amount of dish-washing for small hands."[118] Later, we learn that Frado "was

Household Health in the Domestic's Novel 53

now able to do all the washing, ironing, baking, and the common et cetera of household duties, though but fourteen."[119] Though she matures in age, Frado cannot, it seems, catch up to her chores, which continue to multiply. When Mr. Bellmont remarks to his wife, "The child does as much work as a woman ought to; and just see how she is kicked about!" he marks Frado's overwork as indicative of his wife's failure to recognize her developmental stage and the needs of a "child."[120] By alluding to his wife's horrific physical abuse of her, Mr. Bellmont foreshadows the link between these unreasonable child labor expectations and Frado's future bodily suffering.

In addition to taking on tasks apparently better suited to an adult woman, Frado also performs chores usually reserved for male workers. For instance, she learns from Mrs. Bellmont's son, Jack, how to "drive the cows to pasture," and "in the absence of the men, she must harness the horse for Mary and her mother to ride, go to mill, in short, do the work of a boy, could one be procured to endure the tirades of Mrs. Bellmont."[121] Mrs. Bellmont herself views Frado not as a "bound girl," but as at once "man, boy, housekeeper, domestic, etc."[122] By illustrating the resultant deterioration of Frado's body, Wilson insists on the importance of age and sex to the "physical laws" that nineteenth-century American health reformers championed and the danger of women like Mrs. Bellmont who fail to apply these to the girls working in their homes.

At the same time, Wilson demonstrates that race did not exempt young Black girls from such biological laws. When confronted by her husband for overworking Frado, Mrs. Bellmont insists that African Americans "are just like black snakes; you *can't* kill them. If she wasn't tough she would have been killed long ago. There was never one of my girls could do half the work."[123] Mrs. Bellmont's essentialist explanation for Frado's labor output draws on centuries of white writers' use of biological logic to justify the exploitation of Black women and girls. The purported immunity of Black women to pain during and after childbirth, beginning with falsified sixteenth- and seventeenth-century colonizers' accounts, was seen by slavery's proponents as justifying the violation of feminine norms that their coerced laborer entailed.[124] This belief persisted into the nineteenth century. In 1848, for instance, naturalist Charles Hamilton Smith claimed that "most of the black nations are capable of protracted toil, without much injury to their frames; they willingly share labor with the female sex . . . for many hours, in the tropical sun, without repining."[125] Frado's physical suffering testifies to the fallacy of such racist scientific claims.

As her health breaks down under the weight of her labor, it becomes unsafe for Frado to voice her suffering.[126] For instance, when she is forced to walk barefoot throughout a harsh New England winter that "nearly conquered her physical system," Frado's "complaint[s]" about her lack of protection against the elements are "cruelly punished."[127] Acknowledging her pain to Mrs. Bellmont begets further injury, marking her suffering's disclosure as painful in its own right. Later, too, she becomes "so much reduced as to be unable to stand erect for any great length of time. She would sit at the table to wash her dishes; if she heard the well-known step of her mistress, she would rise till she returned to her room."[128] These efforts to accommodate her ailing body hinder Frado's productivity, which in turn becomes a source of tension between her and those she serves. Eventually, after Frado has turned eighteen and left the Bellmont home, she becomes severely ill and is brought back to the house by members of the community. Unable to accept that Frado is now the expected beneficiary of *her* care, Mrs. Bellmont snaps, "I doubt if she is much sick," a diagnosis that runs counter to that of the doctor who treats her: "you're sick, very sick" he tells Frado, whom he notes is "all broken down" and in need of "good care."[129] Mrs. Bellmont is not only indifferent toward Frado's suffering; her racism prevents her from recognizing Frado's pain as such. Because she believes that Frado *"can't"* become sick, she registers her displays of pain not as involuntary human suffering but as refusals to comply with the racial order of the house.

Frado herself recognizes that "Mrs. Bellmont . . . would have no sympathy for her" amid her illness, and this apathy exacerbates her suffering.[130] At one point, a member of the Bellmont family overhears Frado lamenting to herself, "No one cares for me only to get my work. And I feel sick; who cares for that? Work as long as I can stand, and then fall down and lay there till I can get up. No mother, father, brother or sister to care for me . . . all because I am black! Oh, if I could die!"[131] Frado thrice bemoans not just her overwork but also Mrs. Bellmont's inability to "care" either for her or about her pain, which she marks as a product of her racialization and subsequent classification as "labor power."[132] Frado's physical debilitation, Wilson makes plain, is a product not of her race but rather of others' racism.

After her indenture at the Bellmont home concludes, Frado seeks employment with other local white families. Here, the novel joins *Live and Let Live* in juxtaposing abusive mistresses with those who attend to their domestic workers' health. "Mrs. Moore," for instance, "was a kind friend to her, and attempted to heal her wounded spirit by sympathy and advice, burying the past in the prospects of the future."[133] This concern for her employee's "future," and thus her life (and afterlife) beyond the confines of the home in which she labors, makes Mrs. Moore a clear foil for Mrs. Bellmont. And yet even this benevolent mistress is unable to undo the damage caused by the earlier one. "[Frado's] failing health was a cloud no kindly human hand could dissipate," and she is thus unable to remain in her post.[134] Believing that "they owed her a shelter and attention, when disabled" as compensation for years of labor, she returns to the Bellmonts' home to recuperate.[135] During her stay, Mrs. Bellmont not only refuses to "attend her" herself, which would constitute an inversion of Frado's previous servitude, but also did "not permit her domestic to stay with her at all."[136] While she allows Mr. Bellmont's sister, "Aunt Abby," to nurse Frado until she is well enough to return to Mrs. Moore, Mrs. Bellmont's withholding of aid to her "domestic" frames receiving care as the ultimate signifier of familial belonging.

Frado receives care neither *from* domestics nor *as* a domestic herself. While both Aunt Abby and Mrs. Moore are able to improve her health, neither does so within the framework of an employer caring for a domestic. However, in a letter from the mononymous "Allida" in the novel's appendix that serves as a kind of epilogue, we learn that Frado eventually takes up more sedentary work as a "straw sewer" and, during this time, lived with "Mrs. Walker," a woman whose characterization echoes that of Mrs. Hyde in *Live and Let Live*. Allida quotes a letter from Frado in which she declares that with her new host, "I have at last found a *home*,—and not only a home, but a *mother*."[137] Under the "genial sunshine" of such long-sought maternal care and finally at rest from performing domestic labor, Allida reports that Frado's "health began to improve," and "she even looked forward with *hope*—joyful hope to the future" that Mrs. Bellmont had previously treated as immaterial.[138]

That future, we know from the novel's preface, bears little resemblance to Lucy Lee's happy ending in *Live and Let Live*. On the contrary, the writer (who signs the preface H.E.W. despite the novel's indication of its own authorship as only "by Our Nig") explains that her "failing health" has led her to pen her novel out of economic necessity.[139] Indeed, the novel ends not with a home of Frado's own, but rather with a home for her child. The novel recounts Frado's marriage to Samuel, a Black lecturer on the abolitionist circuit who, in a reenactment of Mag's original abandonment, periodically "desert[s]" Frado and their unnamed son.[140] The affixed letters from both Thorn and Allida recount that, plagued by "poverty and sickness" and "wish[ing] to educate him," Frado, like her mother before her, seeks an alternative home for her child. A far cry from Frado's treatment by the Bellmonts, however, "a kind gentleman and lady took her little boy into their own family, and provided everything necessary for his good."[141] Among this family, her son is not a worker, but rather "he is contented and happy, and . . . considered as good as those he is with."[142]

Frado, too, forges kinship as a result of this arrangement. The family apparently views her child "as one of them, and his mother as a daughter—for they treat her as such" and allow her to visit regularly.[143] The emergence of this familial love amid an otherwise unhappy ending renders the novel an account of disrupted development. While Lucy Lee begins her service as a dependent child and later draws on the health and other domestic knowledge she acquires from her employer to supervise her own home, Frado follows an inverse trajectory. Mrs. Bellmont's exploitation of her youthful vulnerability leaves Frado a dependent *adult* who relies on a benevolent middle-class white family to provide both a home for her son and a familial structure within which she herself is recognized as a surrogate daughter.

Taken together, these domestic's novels illuminate the extent to which race structured the pedagogical relationship between domestics and their employers. While the maternalist care and guidance provided to US-born, white domestics such as Lucy Lee promised a course of maturation that culminated in health and class mobility, the same need for instruction was used to position racialized workers such as Bridget and Frado as fixed in a state of childhood. This, Wilson shows, could have significant physical consequences. In the next chapter, I continue to trace how ideas about physical education shaped the experiences and political ideals of laboring women. I turn to abolitionist writer Harriet Jacobs, whose writing centers on the care work that both free and enslaved Black domestics performed *outside* the middle-class homes in which they labored and beyond the framework of white middle-class maternalism.

CHAPTER THREE

Harriet Jacobs and the Abolitionist "Science of Good Management"

Throughout the decades leading up to the Civil War, abolitionists and defenders of enslavement fiercely debated whether or not African Americans could thrive as free citizens. In the abolitionist press, the phrase "they cannot take care of themselves" stood in for proslavery claims of their dependence on white supervision. In 1841, the *National Anti-Slavery Standard*'s editor, Lydia Maria Child, lamented in the paper that "people are always saying free negroes cannot take care of themselves."[1] An 1843 issue called the claim "stale and ludicrous."[2] Frederick Douglass, too, provided counterevidence in the *North Star*, reporting in 1848 that "many of these runaways who, the slaveholder would have us believe, cannot take care of themselves, are . . . among the most industrious and enterprising of our Northern citizens."[3] "They Cannot Take Care of Themselves" was even the title of an 1842 poem in the *Standard* that mockingly parroted proslavery arguments: "Our Tobacco they plant, and our Cotton they pick; / And our Rice they can harvest and thrash; / They feed us in health, and they nurse us when sick; / And they earn — while we pocket — our cash."[4] While the poem echoes Douglass's emphasis on economic self-sufficiency, the reference to slaves who "nurse us when sick" also suggests another implication of the titular phrase: the domestic labor of caregiving that was a crucial element of physical education.

For Harriet Jacobs, a regular reader of such publications, the poem's critique lay in the reality that for her and many others, providing care was fundamental to enslavement. While chapter 2 showed how ideas about care could be weaponized against racialized women workers, in this chapter, I show how care labor could also be wielded as an abolitionist tool. I recover Jacobs's investment in physical education — which she called "the science of good management" — and argue that she leveraged this expertise to intervene in antebellum debates about African Americans' capacity to "take care of themselves."[5] Jacobs, who performed care labor while enslaved, also worked as a nurse for a white family in the 1850s to support herself and her children while writing *Incidents in the Life of a Slave Girl* (1861). After publishing her narrative, Jacobs volunteered as a "matron" in Civil War "contraband camps" and established schools for formerly enslaved refugees in Virginia and Georgia. Drawing on an archive that includes *Incidents*, her personal and professional correspondence, and her dispatches to the abolitionist press, I show how Jacobs reimagines the labor and discourse of physical education as an abolitionist tool.

Throughout *Incidents* and elsewhere, Jacobs highlights the tensions between enforced labor and forms of self- and community care. In an early scene in *Incidents*, Jacobs's grandmother purchases her uncle's freedom. As mother and son contemplate the future, Jacobs writes that "they would prove to the world that they could take care of themselves, as they had long taken care of others."[6] Koritha Mitchell notes the irony of this passage: the two "had been taking care of themselves all along."[7] In *Incidents* and her other writings, Jacobs shows how African Americans cared for their own bodies and homes, and she clarifies how facilitating fresh air, exercise, and hygiene was essential to physical and psychological well-being.[8] Dorothy Roberts argues that although caring for their families ultimately profited their enslavers, Black women's homemaking was nonetheless a form of resistance.[9] Jacobs shows how such caregiving could also facilitate other forms of dissent. In the decades following her enslavement, caregiving enabled Jacobs to survive while in hiding, fund her abolitionist writing project, and aid other formerly enslaved people.

Although Jacobs's labor approximated that of a "mammy" figure imagined as innately devoted to white children, she supplants such essentialism by highlighting caregiving as a studied scientific field that could be strategically applied.[10] Jacobs would have been well versed in white physical education reformers' ideas about care. Before signing on as Jacobs's editor for *Incidents*, Child had been a prolific author of women's manuals in the 1830s. Unsurprisingly, then, her sole editorial interjection in *Incidents* regards home remedies for a snake bite that Jacobs's pseudonymous protagonist, Linda Brent, suffers.[11] Harriet Beecher Stowe, too, whom Jacobs hoped early on would coauthor her narrative, wrote about domestic instruction with her sister, Catharine Beecher, in 1869, and Jacobs likely read Beecher's earlier works such as the *Treatise* and *Letters* explored in chapter 2.[12] Texts by health reformers were also often reprinted and reviewed in the abolitionist press. In 1849, for instance, while Jacobs was running the Rochester Anti-Slavery Reading Room, Frederick Douglass was in the office directly beneath her, printing health dispatches in the *North Star*.[13]

Across her writings, Jacobs not only exhibits literacy in physical education; she also uses her own caregiving knowledge to intervene in this discourse. Adapting this scientific vernacular into an expressly abolitionist idiom, Jacobs offers a gendered strain of what Britt Rusert terms "fugitive science" in that she "mobilize[s] scientific knowledge in anti-slavery activism."[14] Jacobs performs and records acts of caring for both her own and other African Americans' bodies as expressions of "fugitivity," or what Rusert describes as "a subterranean politics and furtive insurgency against both the Southern slaveholding power and Northern liberalism."[15] Jacobs suggests that if Black women nurses both enslaved and free were expected to bolster the health of white charges, then that expertise could be harnessed in service of Black well-being. Throughout her life, Jacobs both provided and received care. Injured by the effects not only of enslavement but also of her self-emancipation efforts and her labor in the North, Jacobs illustrates the urgency of tending to Black bodies. As historians have demonstrated, enslaved women were often treated as instruments rather than agents of medical knowledge—most infamously in the gynecological experiments Dr. James Marion Sims conducted on Anarcha, Betsey, Lucy, and others in the late 1840s—and Jacobs herself documents the torture she endured by the physician who enslaved her.[16] By turning away from racist medical abuse and toward caregiving as a strategy for resisting enslavement on an individual and collective scale, this chapter traces an alternative, fugitive legacy of enslaved women and health science in the United States.

Racial Science, Slavery, and Care

Proslavery claims of African Americans' dependency on white authority were often grounded in scientific discourses that characterized enslaved people as disabled.[17] One of the most famous treatises on the topic, Dr. Samuel Cartwright's "Report on the Diseases and Physical Peculiarities of the Negro Race" (1851), was first published in the *New Orleans Medical and Surgical Journal* and then reprinted in newspapers across the country, including abolitionist papers. Often cited for inventing such racialized disorders as "drapetomania" (which allegedly drove enslaved people to escape) and "dysaesthesia aethiopis" (a medical explanation for idleness), Cartwright's text also insists that enslaved people were incapable of managing their own bodies.[18] This assertion emerges in a passage Jacobs would have encountered in the *National Anti-Slavery Standard* in March 1853, a few months before her first published work—a letter on the horrors of the slave trade that first appeared in the *New York Tribune*—was reprinted in the *Standard*.[19] The paper quotes Cartwright: "When left to himself, the negro indulges in his natural disposition, idleness and sloth, and does not take exercise enough to expand his lungs and vitalize his blood, but dozes out a miserable existence in the midst of filth and uncleanliness, being too indolent, and having too little energy of mind, to provide for himself proper food and comfortable clothing and lodging."[20] By claiming that African Americans are reluctant to "take exercise enough" on their own accord, Cartwright perversely portrays slave labor as a healthful physical activity.

Cartwright was not alone in this assessment; many argued that enslavement was itself a form of care. Josiah Clark Nott and George R. Gliddon's *Types of Mankind* (1854) propagated Samuel Morton's assertion that "the Negro thrives under the shadow of his white master . . . and exists and multiplies in increased physical well-being."[21] In 1858, Thomas R. R. Cobb similarly proposed that as a result of bondage, African Americans' "physical development is unquestionably much superior to that of the negro in his native country."[22] However, the abilities of African American women in particular are an implicit concern in Cartwright's account. Cartwright makes no gender distinctions in the excerpt reprinted in the *Standard*, employing exclusively masculine pronouns to describe the entire population of enslaved people. However, his invocation of domestic responsibilities related to hygiene, diet, and clothing as health determinants reveals the significance of feminized labor to Cartwright's theory. His circular logic suggests that African American (women's) innately "indolent" disposition renders them incapable of domestic management, which in turn explains their physical inferiority.

Race scientists had to reckon, however, with the reality that African American women did provide care and that such labor was often essential to their "value" as property. In 1848, Charles Hamilton Smith argued that in "black nations," "the female sex is affectionate, to absolute devotedness, in the character of mother, child, nurse, and attendant upon the sick . . . as housewives, they are charitable to the wants of the wayfaring visitants; within doors orderly; and, personally, very clean."[23] This position was quickly overshadowed by arguments that such a propensity for domestic labor was not innate in Black women but rather produced through what Morton called the "strong powers of imitation" that suited them to "mechanic arts."[24] Indeed, in an 1858 treatise, disdainfully excerpted in *The Liberator* that same year, Cartwright addressed the subject of Black women's caregiving directly: "Nor will the women undress the children and put them regularly to bed. . . . They let their children suffer and die, or unmercifully abuse them, unless the white man or woman prescribes rules in the nursery for them to go by."[25]

In *Incidents*, Jacobs provides horrific counterevidence to Cartwright's suggestion that white women were superior caregivers. The home in *Incidents* is not simply a site of feminine authority; it also houses the violence of white domestic structures.[26] Jacobs writes that Brent's enslaver, "Mrs. Flint, like many southern women, was totally deficient in energy. She had not strength to superintend her household affairs; but her nerves were so strong, that she could sit in her easy chair and see a woman whipped, till the blood trickled from every stroke of the lash."[27] As Hazel Carby has shown, this passage reveals the "Southern lady" as "a corrupt and superficial veneer that covers an underlying strength and power in cruelty and brutality."[28] Jacobs's critique also channels abolitionist ideas about Southern domesticity. Her account of Mrs. Flint echoes Child's claim in *The History of the Condition of Women, in Various Ages and Nations* (1835) that "the southern ladies [of the United States] are delicately formed, with pale complexions, a languid gracefulness of manner, and a certain aristocratic bearing, acquired only by the early habit of commanding those who are deemed immeasurably inferior."[29] This characterization also invokes one of the texts held in the Rochester Anti-Slavery Reading Room: George Bourne's *Slavery Illustrated in Its Effects upon Woman and Domestic Society* (1837). Decreeing slavery physically detrimental to white women, Bourne claims that the typical Southern woman is "a puny, debilitated and almost helpless creature" whose "body is as feeble as her mind is enervated" and lacks crucial "physical energies."[30] Jacobs's reference to Mrs. Flint's avoidance of "household affairs," however, entrenches her critique in discourses of domestic labor. In the same passage she writes, "She would station herself in the kitchen, and wait till [dinner] was dished, and then spit in all the kettles and pans that had been used for cooking. She did this to prevent the cook and her children from eking out their meagre fare with the remains."[31] Mrs. Flint is not only removed from the work that occurs in the kitchen but actually inverts this arena of care labor by rendering it a site of deprivation and physical harm.

Beyond the kitchen, Jacobs shows how caregiving responsibilities put enslaved women in danger, most powerfully through the figure of Aunt Nancy, who "was housekeeper and waiting-maid in Dr. Flint's family. Indeed, she was the *factotum* of the household. Nothing went on well without her."[32] Her treatment by Mrs. Flint illustrates how white women abused those they entrusted with caring for their children: "expecting to be a mother," she requires Aunt Nancy to "lie at her door" in case "she should want a drink of water in the night."[33] Aunt Nancy, pregnant herself, miscarries because of the strain. Later, when Mrs. Flint's child was born, Aunt Nancy "was required to resume her place on the entry floor, because Mrs. Flint's babe needed her attentions. She kept her station there through the summer and winter, until she had given premature birth to six children; and all the while she was employed as night-nurse to Mr. Flint's children."[34] The demands of caring for the Flints' (unborn) white child injure Aunt Nancy and prevent her from becoming a mother herself. The scene ultimately reflects Jacobs's claim earlier in her narrative that "my mistress, like many others, seemed to think that slaves had no right to any family ties of their own; that they were created merely to wait upon the family of the mistress."[35]

Jacobs also describes (via Brent) the abuse that she herself endured as a caregiver in the Flint home. In fact, one of the most vivid accounts of their cruelty directly contrasts the concerns about domestic workers that Child articulates in *The Mother's Book* (1831). Though far less focused than Beecher on domestic workers' supposed failings, Child nonetheless worried about their moral influence. "It is a bad plan for young girls to sleep with nursery maids," she warns her readers. "There is a strong love among vulgar people of telling secrets, and talking on forbidden subjects."[36] Because of this vulgarity, she continues, "a prudent mother will very rarely . . . place her daughter in the same sleeping apartment with a domestic."[37] Such nursing responsibility made Jacobs vulnerable to sexual abuse. She recalls an evening when Dr. Flint, who had long "whisper[ed] foul words in my ear" and "peopled my young mind with unclean images," "announced his intention to take his youngest daughter, then four years old, to sleep in his apartment," bringing Brent along "to be on hand if the child stirred."[38] Aware of her husband's intentions, Mrs. Flint intervenes—though not out of concern for Brent. On the contrary, "she now took me to sleep in a room adjoining her own," where "I was an object of her especial care."[39] Jacobs quickly clarifies the irony of such "care," writing that, at night, Mrs. Flint "whispered in my ear, as though it was her husband who was speaking to me."[40] She is not only "corrupted" by her enslaver but made "fearful for my life," which "had often been threatened" on such nights.[41] While Child feared that nurses would damage their white charges, Jacobs shows how domestic arrangements made Black nurses physically and psychologically vulnerable.

Both Aunt Nancy's and Brent's impairments represent what Dennis Tyler calls "racial injury," a particular mode of psychological and physical disablement that nineteenth-century African American authors and activists documented. In doing so, they refused the figuration of disability as an inherent feature of Blackness by white writers such as Cartwright, Nott, and Gliddon.[42] Jacobs's extended portrayal of the ways Mrs. Flint harms the women she enslaves illuminates a gendered form of such imposed impairment. The domestic responsibility for others' health, *Incidents* makes clear, created a unique site of racial injury that paradoxically played out within the context of care.

Self-Care and Survival in *Incidents*

Domestic spaces are central not only to Brent's enslavement but also to Jacobs's construction of fugitivity. As Valerie Smith observes, enclosures both figurative and literal pervade Jacobs's narrative.[43] Evading Dr. Flint, Brent hides in the attic, beneath the floorboards in a friend's mistress's home, and in a nine-by-seven-by-three-foot garret in her grandmother's house for seven years. These hyperbolically confining domestic spaces are sites of caregiving, though here it is Brent's own body, rather than those of white children, that becomes the object of care. Domestic manuals often encouraged mothers to tend to their own bodies to facilitate their labor. While, as Carby argues, Jacobs's narrative reveals the false promise of "True Womanhood's" insistence on purity and submissiveness, she also critiques a model that dominated reform ideology: what Frances Cogan calls "Real Womanhood," which privileged physical capacity and industriousness.[44] According to Diane Price Herndl, Jacobs extends this discourse to African American women such as Brent's grandmother and Aunt Nancy, but ultimately critiques "Real Womanhood's" failure to address the exhausting, injurious demands placed on working-class women.[45] Perhaps the most salient dimension of Jacobs's critique of this discourse, however, lies in her politicization of the health practices associated with it.

Although critics have proposed that Jacobs minimizes Brent's physical suffering while in hiding to combat the perception of Black women as hyperembodied, her turn to domestic scientific methods suggests that she manages, rather than ignores, her injuries.[46] Brent's (and Jacobs's) diligent attention to her embodiment reflects an important tenet of domestic management. In *The Mother's Book*, Child explains, "A mother needs to be something of a philosopher. — In other, and better words, she needs a great deal of practical good sense, and habits of close observation."[47] Brent emerges as just such an observer in the garret. In addition to her surveillance of Dr. Flint and others through a peephole, she keeps watch over her own body. The first observation Jacobs records upon Brent's confinement is that the "air was stifling."[48] She displays careful attention to her bodily experience, noting, "it seemed horrible to sit or lie in a cramped position day after day."[49] As the narrative progresses, Jacobs reports that Brent "longed to draw in a plentiful draught of fresh air, to stretch my cramped limbs, to have room to stand erect, to feel the earth under my feet again."[50] As her observations shift to imagined remedies, Jacobs underscores Brent's health knowledge and portrays her coerced confinement as a barrier to enacting self-care.

Of Brent's manifold physical deprivations in the garret, Jacobs underscores two in particular, air and mobility: "I lived in that little dismal hole, almost deprived of light and air, and with no space to move my limbs, for nearly seven years."[51] As Mary Titus suggests, these related needs likely appealed to Jacobs rhetorically for their "mixing of medical prescription with physical liberation."[52] These concerns also put Brent's health knowledge in conversation with domestic advice. "It is strange," muses the author of an 1849 entry in the *North Star*, "that so many American women can submit to be cooped up day after day, week after week, in a confined room . . . scarcely ever once in a month breathing a mouthful of fresh air, or taking five minutes' healthful exercise. . . . How can nervous and delicate women expect to endure it?"[53] Another 1849 entry entitled "Exercise," too, insisted that "open air" and "daily fatigue" would promote "healthy feelings and good looks."[54] In 1853, while Jacobs was working on *Incidents*, the newspaper (by then renamed *Frederick Douglass' Paper*) ran an article entitled "Fresh Air" that implored readers to "open your windows—let in the fresh air" for the sake of their health.[55] Child, too instructed women to "sleep in rooms with a free circulation of air" and take "exercise in the open air" in order to cultivate health.[56]

Though her access to "fresh air" is limited by her confinement to the garret, Brent does pursue physical exercise, directly contesting Cartwright's assertion that "the negro . . . does not take exercise" without supervision.[57] Although "it was impossible . . . to move in an erect position," Brent adapts her movements: "I crawled about my den for exercise."[58] It is during one such exertion, in fact, that she makes a crucial discovery. "One day" while crawling, Brent "hit [her] head against something, and found it was a gimlet," which she then used to bore a hole through which to observe her children, a development that Jacobs reports provides some "consolation" and "pleasure."[59] Here the pursuit of exercise links Brent's physical health to her psychological well-being, as well as her maternal identity. Counter to Cartwright's claims, her concern for her own health actually facilitates her keeping watch over her children—itself a form of care.

Such scenes of pursuing health practices under injurious conditions also refute assertions of the Black female body's capacity to endure pain.

Allegations of Black women's inherently elevated endurance were used to construct them as physiologically other and justify the violation of feminine norms that their forced labor entailed.[60] Narrating Brent's ability to withstand the extreme conditions of her concealment thus poses a problem for Jacobs in that it risks corroborating such racist scientific claims. At the same time, while associations of frailty with femininity made illness a possible means of either sexual identification with white readers or, as Saidiya V. Hartman argues, an instrumentalized spectacle of suffering, notions of Black corporeality as itself impairment also made displays of disability fraught.[61] Jacobs, however, circumvents this "problem of embodiment" by turning to domestic science.[62] She depicts impairment not only as something that happens to Black bodies when under duress but also as an event to which she is expertly equipped to respond.

Brent's efforts to exercise while in hiding are not, however, entirely successful, and Jacobs underscores the persistence of impairment despite Brent's interventions. As Dea H. Boster has shown, disability did not hinder people from fleeing enslavement, and *Incidents* reveals the role of health *practices*, rather than an idealized healthy body, in facilitating such resistance.[63] Once again presenting Brent as knowledgeable about her own health, Jacobs writes that her "grandmother began to listen to my entreaty to be allowed to leave my cell, sometimes, and exercise my limbs to prevent my becoming a cripple."[64] The implication that such movements will counter the impairments produced by Brent's confinement is, however, quickly undermined. Her efforts "to bring warmth and feeling into my limbs" are "without avail," and she remains "so numb and stiff that it was a painful effort to move."[65]

Her efforts are also risky, and Jacobs writes that "had my enemies come upon me during the first mornings I tried to exercise them a little in the small unoccupied space of the storeroom, it would have been impossible for me to have escaped."[66] This reflection echoes an earlier scene in which Brent's Uncle Benjamin becomes ill while hiding in the North: "His strength was slow in returning; and his desire to continue his journey seemed to retard his recovery. How could he get strength without air and exercise?"[67] When he finally ventures out, he encounters a white acquaintance from the South. Though he leaves the interaction unscathed, the scene underscores the problem posed not only by impairment but also by efforts to recover from it. Both Brent and Benjamin are confronted with a paradox: outdoor exercise may facilitate the mobility "running away" demands, but it is also untenable, given the imperative to remain hidden.

This tension is further complicated by Jacobs's suggestion that attending to her health is key not only to Brent's escape from the South but also to her subsistence in the North. When the opportunity finally arises to leave the garret, Brent responds in terms of her body's limited capacity: "The anticipation of being a free woman proved almost too much for my weak frame."[68] Freedom, it seems, requires a degree of physical preparation made impossible by the conditions of Brent's hiding place and their effect on her health. And yet the "excitement" of her impending departure only "almost" overwhelms her and instead "stimulate[s]" her to make "busy preparations" for the journey.[69] The promise of freedom is thus itself a physically animating force that is, as the unfolding narrative confirms, incompatible with Brent's lingering impairments.

Brent's relocation to the North in *Incidents* marks an important shift in the narrative's treatment of health and caregiving. Before she leaves, Brent's grandmother offers her money, explaining, "You may be sick among strangers . . . and they would send you to the poorhouse to die."[70] Jacobs's ability to support herself financially was indeed dependent on managing her health. Despite Jacobs's claims in *Incidents* that "constant exercise on board the vessel" headed to Philadelphia "and frequent rubbing with salt water, had nearly restored the use of my limbs," Brent continues to experience mobility impairments while seeking employment in the North.[71] The abolitionist Joshua Coffin reported to Child in 1842, the year of Jacobs's escape, that "she has been shut up so long that she can hardly walk."[72] Jacobs corroborates this account, describing Brent's first days in the North: "My greatest anxiety now was to obtain employment. My health was greatly improved, though my limbs continued to trouble me with swelling whenever I walked much."[73]

Abolitionists posited that the conditions of freedom would not only alleviate African American's impairments, but also that such rehabilitation would facilitate their self-sufficiency. For example, Child's *An Appeal in Favor of That Class of Americans Called Africans* (1833) includes an excerpt from Harriet Martineau's *Illustrations of Political Economy: Demerara*, published the previous year: "Where a man is allowed the possession of himself, the purchaser of his labor is benefitted by the vigor of his mind through the service of his limbs: where man is made the possession of another, the possessor loses at once and for ever all that is most valuable in that for which he has paid the price of crime."[74] Martineau's claim that slavery devalues labor depends on the presumption that free laborers have control of their "limbs"—the very site of Brent's impairment. The description of able-bodied labor as more "valuable" recalls the discourse of "soundness" that structured medical and legal interpretations of enslaved people's market value. These resonances underscore the limitations posed by abolitionist assumptions of able-bodied labor under freedom.[75] This dynamic is explicated in Jacobs's narrative by the fact that her potentially disqualifying impairments are the direct result of her escape. The explicit connection she draws between her ongoing injury and her employment suggests that the physical effects of her self-emancipation undermine the promise of able-bodied self-sufficiency so central to abolitionist rhetoric.

When Brent does find employment as a baby nurse for "Mrs. Bruce" (a pseudonym for Mary Stace Willis, who hired Jacobs in 1842), she draws on her previously self-sustaining health knowledge to perform domestic labor that ultimately injures her own body. While women described as "mammies" were assumed to possess exceptional physical ability that contrasted the delicacy of their white charges, Jacobs highlights her own physical precarity in this role.[76] Her work exacerbates her impairments: "The necessity of passing up and down stairs frequently, caused my limbs to swell so painfully . . . I became unable to perform my duties."[77] Virginia Cope has described the trajectory of *Incidents* as "a journey from a pre-capitalist South into a free-labor North" that culminates in her disillusionment with capitalism.[78] If, as Cope suggests, Brent imagines her entrance into this economy in terms of her ability to sell her labor, the lingering corporeal effects of her escape pose an important critique of this false promise of autonomy.[79]

Brent's care labor also renders her physically unsafe. As Brent senses the tenuousness of her freedom, Jacobs depicts scenes of childcare with a sense of terror. She describes feeling "haunted" when "it was necessary for me to take little Mary out daily, for exercise and fresh air" because she fears that someone "might recognize me."[80] This feeling intensifies after the passage of the Fugitive Slave Act in 1850, which renders caregiving dangerous. "All that winter," Jacobs writes, "I lived in a state of anxiety. When I took the children out to breathe the air, I closely observed the countenances of all I met."[81] The "exercise and fresh air" she had pursued intently while in hiding emerge now as a threat to her freedom and well-being, rather than a boon to her health.

At the conclusion of *Incidents*, after Brent's first employer has died and her husband remarries, the second "Mrs. Bruce" (Cornelia Grinnell Willis) purchases Brent's freedom. Her fugitive status, however, persists. Because of the demands of her work and the proslavery views of her employer, Nathaniel Parker Willis, she composed her narrative largely in secret, "whenever [she] could snatch an hour from household duties."[82] In 1853, she moved with the Willis family to Idlewild, their home upstate in Cornwall, where Willis believed the climate would improve his family's health. At the same time that Jacobs was writing *Incidents*, Willis was composing *Out-Doors at Idlewild* (1855), in which he declared that "nine out of ten of the medicines for every disease are prescribed by Nature—fresh air, exercise, control of habits and appetite, etc."[83] Jacobs is mentioned only briefly as "my daughter's nurse, who has had the care of all her bright eleven years, having been . . . a slave."[84] When Willis asserts that "confinement to the regulated temperature of a room, in any latitude, is certain death," he was surely unaware that, elsewhere on the property, Jacobs was recounting just such a near-death experience: describing an illness Brent suffered in the garret, Jacobs writes that, under the advice of a "Thompsonian doctor," her brother made her a fire, "but there was no outlet for the gas, and it nearly cost me my life."[85]

Jacobs was not only recounting illness while at Idlewild; she was also experiencing it. Her letters to Amy Kirby Post, a Rochester Ladies Anti-Slavery Society member with whom she had lived during her year in Rochester, reveal that her labor threatened to impede her health as well as her writing project. In addition to the lingering mobility impairments documented in *Incidents*, Jacobs reports "Rheumatism," "a Tumer [sic] on my womb," and "congestion of the lungs."[86] Her correspondence shows how the demands of nursing paradoxically leave little opportunity to tend to her own health as she had in hiding. In July 1854, for instance, she details a doctor's prescription that she "give up five Months [sic] and he can cure," but, by December, Jacobs was still at work and continued to "suffer very much from my left side."[87] By the following summer, when she was diagnosed with a tumor, she began to consider a link between her employment and her illness, reporting to Post, "I can never get well while I am at a service."[88]

The threats to her health and her abolitionist writing project were also related. In a March 1854 letter to Post, Jacobs apologizes for her delayed correspondence, explaining, "When I would have written I was in Bed with a severe attack of Rheumatism so that I could not raise my hands to my head, I am still suffering with it in my shoulders."[89] Jacobs's illness directly disrupts her writing process, imparting new, material meaning to other embodied authorial moments in *Incidents*. Expressing a desire for "more ability" in furthering the abolitionist cause, Jacobs laments, "My heart is so full, and my pen is so weak!"[90] Furthermore, when she reports toward the end of *Incidents* that "it has been painful to me, in many ways, to recall the dreary years I passed in bondage," she refers perhaps not only to revisiting traumatic memories but also to the physical pain that the act of writing occasions.[91]

When, in 1857, Jacobs asked Post to write a preface to *Incidents*, she implored her to "mention that I lived at service all the while that I was striving to get the Book out," as she did not want "to have people think that I was living an Idle life—and had to get this book out merely to make money."[92] By capitalizing "Idle," she alludes to her location while also distancing herself from it—her "service" at Idlewild is a far cry from the restorative reprieve her employers sought, but rather a period of politically urgent, painful composition.

Care among the Contrabands

After the successful publication of *Incidents*, caregiving emerges for Jacobs as a more explicitly antislavery tool. While her work for the Willis family often impeded both her health and her abolitionist efforts, Jacobs later found an opportunity to apply her caregiving expertise to her activism. With the commencement of the Civil War, roughly 500,000 African Americans fled enslavement, and many converged on the nation's capital, forming refugee camps where Union officials referred to them as "contraband" and struggled to provide them with adequate housing and care.[93] Jim Downs has shown how this refugee crisis gave way to widespread sickness and death.[94] Northern volunteers who traveled to the earliest camps, intending to dispense Christian education, discovered rampant illness caused by crowded living conditions and inadequate supplies. Their focus quickly shifted to a comprehensive emphasis on health that, for women volunteers, involved applying domestic scientific knowledge to prevent the further spread of disease.

In 1862, Jacobs traveled to Washington, DC, as an agent of the New York Yearly Meeting of the Society of Friends. She tended to refugees there and in nearby Alexandria, Virginia, until shortly after the formation of the Freedmen's Bureau in the spring of 1865, when she relocated to Savannah, Georgia, to continue her relief efforts. According to Child, Jacobs spent these years "comforting the afflicted, nursing the sick, and teaching the children."[95] Federal and military agency reports on the "contraband camps" often minimized the widespread sickness among the refugees in favor a triumphant narrative that equated freedom with health.[96] Northern reformers were thus the primary documentarians of the deprivations formerly enslaved people faced, and Jacobs wrote regularly about her relief work both in her personal correspondence and in dispatches to Northern philanthropic organizations and the abolitionist press.

Jacobs drew on her health knowledge extensively in her reports from the camps, where she encountered refugees "without bedding, without a change of clothing, without nourishment, without the commonest necessaries for the comfort of the sick and dying."[97] Her earliest and most extensive account, "Life among the Contrabands," appeared in *The Liberator* on September 5, 1862, as a letter addressed to the editor, William Lloyd Garrison. In this report, the oscillations between stasis and exercise that structure her narration of the garret reemerge when she juxtaposes unhygienic facilities to more healthful conditions. Of the refugees at Duff Green's Row in Washington, she writes, "Some of them were in the most pitiable condition. Many were sick with measles, diptheria [sic], scarlet and typhoid fever. Some had a few filthy rags to lie on; others had nothing but the bare floor for a couch."[98] At the spacious Union-occupied property in Arlington Heights, however, the conditions were far better. "At the quarters," she reports, "there are many contrabands. The men are employed, and most of the women. Here they have plenty of exercise in the open air, and seem very happy."[99] As in *Incidents*, Jacobs underscores the related importance of both bodily exertion and fresh air. A far cry from Washington's unhygienic, crowded facilities, Jacobs frames the conditions at Arlington Heights as ideal partly because they are conducive to health.

Jacobs's efforts were part of a larger philanthropic apparatus that was dominated by white women. With the formation of the camps, the debate about Black dependency on white slaveholders extended to concerns that refugees were overly reliant on white aid. Proslavery advocates argued that widespread illness was evidence that African Americans were better off under slavery.[100] In contrast, reformers including Jacobs urgently worked to alleviate suffering and equip refugee women with domestic health knowledge. After years of writing manuals for white women, for example, Child explained to the formerly enslaved readership of *The Freedmen's Book* (1865) that "there are three things peculiarly essential to health, —plenty of fresh water, plenty of pure air, and enough of nourishing food."[101] Margaret Geneva Long suggests that by emphasizing domestic labor as requisite to their thriving as free women, aid workers imposed their own normative constructions of femininity on the refugees.[102] By providing such physical education training, volunteers strangely implied that formerly enslaved women had no previous knowledge of such labor. Jacobs's own writing espoused this maternalist ideology. In "Life among the Contrabands," she laments that "there was no matron in the house" at Duff Green's Row, "and nothing at hand to administer to the comfort of the sick and dying."[103] Jacobs, who would be appointed "matron" of a similar camp in Alexandria the following year, regularly documented the "improvement" she observed in the refugees under her care.[104] When Jacobs left Virginia to continue her relief work in Georgia, she explained her decision in terms that invoked earlier abolitionist articulations, writing in an 1865 report: "The freed people here, with but a small exception, can now take care of themselves."[105]

Jacobs's relief work itself was often treated by white reformers as evidence of African Americans' capacity for self-management. In a preface to "Colored Refugees in Our Camps," a letter from Jacobs published in *The Liberator* in 1863, Child reports that she has been "manifesting sympathy with her long-oppressed people by nursing them in the vicinity of our camps. To do this, she not only relinquishes good wages in a family for many years strongly attached to her, but also liberally imparts from her own earnings to the destitute around her."[106] Linking her work for the Willis family to her current post, Child implicitly identifies Jacobs as an experienced, skilled nurse. Child's reference to Jacobs acting on behalf of the "destitute" also invokes her instructions in *The Family Nurse* (1837), in which she claims that philanthropy is itself healthful: "A walk in connexion [sic] with active business, or to relieve the necessities of the *destitute*, is worth ten walks merely for exercise."[107] Jacobs's relief work, by this logic, is a way of caring for herself in that it benefits her own body as well as those of others.

Child also identifies Jacobs as "a very worthy, intelligent woman, who was herself a slave during twenty-five years," highlighting her trajectory from enslavement to reformer.[108] An 1865 report in the *Freedmen's Record* further underscores Jacobs's own "improvement," declaring that "this slave girl is now one of the most zealous and efficient workers in the Freedmen's cause."[109] Though "all her energies were exhausted in caring for [the refugees'] physical needs," Jacobs has, by this account, "been unwearied in her labors, in providing orphan children with homes, in nursing the sick, in assisting the able-bodied to find work, and in encouraging all in habits of industry and self-reliance."[110] Crystal S. Donkor has noted that Jacobs's correspondence, too, suggests that her "health," in Jacobs's words, "[was] better than it had been for years," and that this recovery suggests that finding "a different cause for which to labor" alleviated much of her suffering.[111] The lingering impairments that once threatened to hinder Jacobs from composing *Incidents* are nowhere to be found. Rather, Jacobs emerges as reformers' ideal woman: both remarkably vigorous and capable of cultivating this quality in others.

Jacobs understood her relief work as distinctly gendered. In addition to performing feminized care labor, she focused specifically on aiding women. In the opening paragraph of "Life among the Contrabands," she reports, "I found men, women and children all huddled together, without any distinction or regard to age or sex."[112] This depiction, published only weeks prior to the Emancipation Proclamation, resonates with what Hortense Spillers describes as the "undifferentiated identity" imposed on captured Africans by the horrors of the Middle Passage and enslavement.[113] Encountering the refugees as a singular mass, Jacobs invokes the "ungendered" flesh that Spillers argues was produced in the starkly antidomestic space of the slave ship's crowded hold.[114] In her reading of Spillers, Nirmala Erevelles suggests that the transformation of the socially demarcated "body" into "ungendered" "flesh" is produced partly by the "imbrication of blackness and disability."[115] Jacobs makes a similar move, describing the refugees' impairments as exacerbated by the same conditions that impede sex differentiation. "Many of them," she reports, "suffer much from the confinement in this crowded building. . . . It is almost impossible to keep the building in a healthy condition."[116] She later reports optimistically that "a new Superintendent was engaged" who "went to work in earnest pulling down partitions to enlarge the rooms, that he might establish two hospitals, one for the men and another for the women."[117] The reinstatement of sex difference, she suggests, is prerequisite to health care.

Jacobs worked extensively to provide women refugees with physical education. In 1863, for instance, she formed "a large sewing circle, composed of young and old" in Alexandria.[118] Jacobs also played a crucial rule in health education among African Americans. "In the school-room," Jacobs reports in "Life among the Contrabands," "I could not but feel how much these young women and children needed female teachers who could do something more than teach them their A, B, C. They need to be taught the right habits of living and the true principles of life."[119] Echoing her account of the superintendent in Alexandria, Jacobs imagines education as a way of reinstating the markers of sex difference eradicated by inhospitable living conditions. Women, she suggests, should teach women, because of their shared domestic concerns, those "habits of living" she deems crucial to well-being.

Jacobs's caring for other Black women in the camps complicates the racial politics of relief work. Although white women reformers sought to convey African Americans' capacity for independence, their efforts also risked corroborating Beecher's claim two decades earlier that "the lower classes" required Anglo-American supervision in domestic work. As a Black woman relief worker, Jacobs unsettled this paradigm, and she was not the only one to do so. In 1862, the writer and personal dressmaker to Mary Todd Lincoln, Elizabeth Keckley, founded the Contraband Relief Association after asking herself, "If the white people can give festivals to raise funds for the relief of suffering soldiers, why should not the well-to-do colored people go to work to do something for the benefit of the suffering blacks?"[120] A decade later, abolitionist and educator Maria W. Stewart served as matron of the Freedmen's Hospital in Washington, DC, where she also established a religious school for "poor and destitute children."[121] Jacobs's writings from her own matron post illuminate how Black women's relief efforts destabilized the maternalism of their white counterparts. Though Jacobs often signaled her affiliation with white abolitionists by reporting on the refugees' ability to "take care of themselves," she also makes a crucial revision to this recognizable phrase. In "Life among the Contrabands," she implores readers to "trust [the refugees], make them free, and give them the responsibility of caring for themselves, and they will soon learn to help *each other*."[122] For Jacobs, relief work is not simply about forming discrete domestic familial arrangements with women at the helm; it is also about establishing caregiving as a collective concern.

This commitment recalls scenes throughout *Incidents* when Brent, so often a caregiver herself, receives care from other enslaved people. When she is bitten by a snake while in hiding, for example, Brent and a friend treat the wound with a "poultice of warm ashes and vinegar" before consulting "an old woman, who doctored among the slaves" and applying her prescription of "cankered vinegar."[123] Similarly, while hidden in the garret, Brent describes her brother retrieving "herbs, roots, and ointment" from a "Thompsonian doctor."[124] She receives physical education instruction too, before she takes cover in the garret. Her friend, Peter, provides one final prescription before her long incarceration that seems to have shaped her attention to self-care: "You must make the most of this walk," he tells her, "for you may not have another very soon."[125] This collaborative approach to health shapes Jacobs's relief work during the war. Much like Douglass's matter-of-factly reprinted health advice in the *North Star*, Jacobs takes the physical education knowledge that has long been available to networks of white homemakers and disseminates it among African American women. Although her work with white Northern reformers might situate her within a maternalist project, Jacobs's educational efforts also sow the seeds of a community-based approach to health.

Jacobs's writings establish caregiving as a strategy of what Mitchell terms "homemade citizenship," or a sense of belonging and success that exists independent of national recognition. "African Americans," Mitchell explains, "keep embracing everything associated with the ideal citizen, including . . . traditional homemaking," even though "they know their accomplishments will more likely inspire attack than respectability and safety."[126] In "Colored Refugees in Our Camps," Jacobs signals the necessity of valuing Black caregiving beyond a move toward national inclusion in her description of Union soldiers arriving at a Virginia camp: "The colored people could not do enough for the first regiments that came here . . . the sight of the U.S. uniform . . . inspired them with hope and confidence. Many of them freely fed the soldiers at their own tables, and lodged them as comfortable as possible in their humble dwellings."[127] Dressed in "the U.S. uniform," these soldiers represent the nation itself. Rather than require their aid, the refugees attempt to care *for* the soldiers, thus signaling their membership in the national community of which they are presumably part. "In return for their kindness and ever-ready service," however, Jacobs reports of the refugees, "they often receive insults, and sometimes beatings, and so they have learned to distrust those who wear the uniform of the U.S."[128] The performance of caregiving is met with what Mitchell calls "know-your-place aggression" that demonstrates the limitations of white frameworks of national belonging.[129]

Importantly, Jacobs records the Union army's violence toward the refugees in 1863, relatively early in her relief work and before she began establishing schools. Jacobs's turn to education signals the importance of constructing new institutions that operate outside the existing structures that the abusive Union army represents. If, as Mitchell argues, Brent "defines accomplishment in relation to homemaking" in *Incidents*, then Jacobs's relief work extends this definition by enmeshing her domestic successes with those of other Black women.[130] Jacobs eventually opened two schools where refugees studied what she called "the right habits of living."[131] With her daughter, Louisa (Ellen in *Incidents*), she founded the Jacobs School in Virginia in 1864 and the Lincoln School in Georgia in 1865. Though not a teacher herself, Jacobs saw herself as an educator. In 1865, she wrote that the refugees "at one time thought me very hard, for I was always preaching to them about taking care of themselves; some would feel it was right, and act accordingly; others, that my only duty was to clothe their bodies; but they do not think so now, for many of them have learned that self-reliance is the elevation of their race."[132] Jacobs draws a clear line between two distinct

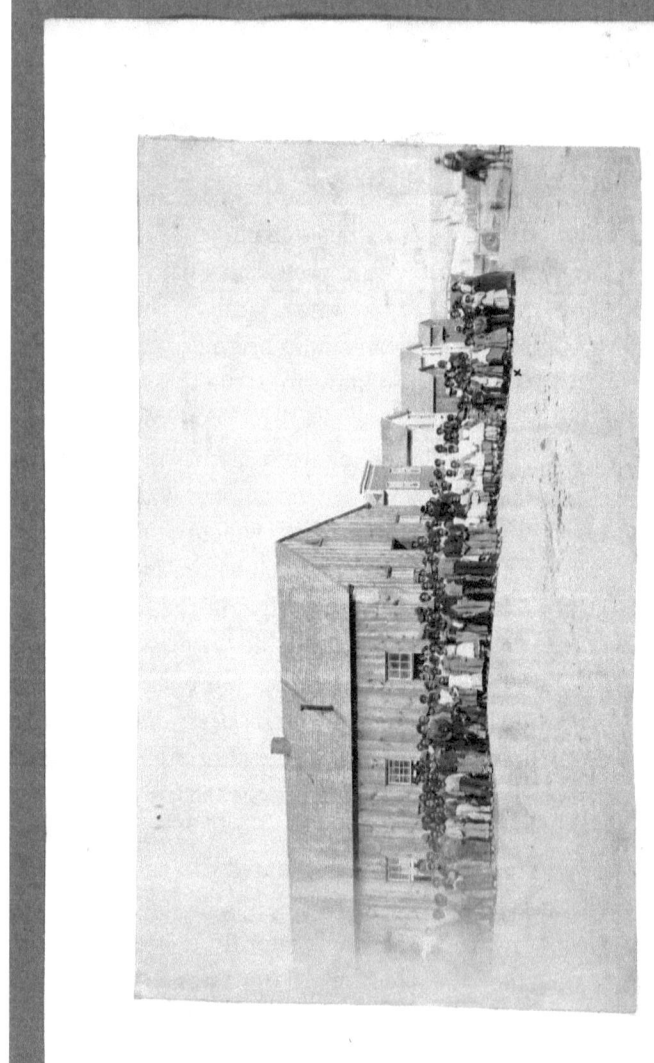

Teachers and pupils of the Jacobs School in Alexandria, Virginia, 1864. Jacobs's face is visible behind the children under whom an "x" has been drawn. Robert Langmuir African American photograph collection, circa 1840–2000. Courtesy of Emory University, Stuart A. Rose Manuscript, Archives, and Rare Book Library.

forms of care here: she is not there only to administer direct care by "cloth[ing] their bodies"—she aims to teach such caregiving skills. Jacobs saw value in Black women providing such instruction. In an 1864 letter, she writes of her newly established school in Virginia, "I do not object to a white teacher . . . but I think it has a good effect upon these people to convince them that their own race can do something for their Elevation. . . . It inspires them with confidence to help each other."[133]

Jacobs's daughter became exactly the kind of Black teacher she describes here. Louisa had been educated in the late 1840s at Hiram H. Kellogg's predominantly white Young Ladies' Domestic Seminary in Clinton, New York, where she was trained in academic subjects as well as exposed to a physical education curriculum that included housework, cooking, nursing, and sewing.[134] These became crucial to her pedagogy, and she taught domestic sciences in "industrial departments" for women and children in her mother's schools and later in a similar department at Howard University.[135] Such training, according to another teacher's letter published in the *Freedmen's Record* a year after the Jacobs School was founded, involved "sewing and its accompaniments," but it also sought to instill domestic values by "teach[ing] . . . mothers and wives how to live good lives, and how to make a happy, social, and virtuous home."[136]

The curriculum that Jacobs imagines and that her daughter enacts is remarkably similar to those described in Black abolitionist Frances Ellen Watkins Harper's 1892 novel, *Iola Leroy, or Shadows Uplifted*, which follows a Black woman's relief efforts during the Civil War and Reconstruction. Harper, who lectured on behalf of equal rights with Louisa during the latter's brief 1867 stint as a lecturer in New York, portrays her heroine serving first (like Jacobs) as a nurse and later (like Louisa) as a teacher among formerly enslaved refugees.[137] Harper writes that Iola's "school was beginning to lift up the home, for Iola was not satisfied to teach her children only the rudiments of knowledge. She had tried to lay the foundation of good character."[138] Later in the novel, too, Iola teaches at a school for African American women designed specifically "to train future wives and mothers."[139] The school here, as in Jacobs's account, becomes a site of domestic preparation, directly influencing "the home." Though focused on preparing young women to manage their homes, Louisa's industrial departments were housed in sites that overlapped with those of health care. In Savannah, the school was housed in the newly established hospital. As Louisa wrote in 1866, "My school-room is in one of the wards portioned off. . . . My room is rough, but large and airy."[140] Her teaching became health care in part by proximity; Louisa worked alongside nurses in her "ward" of the hospital. The health concerns about "air" that pervade her mother's earlier writing, too, appear in Louisa's description, revealing her responsibility for students' physical as well as mental development.

While Louisa was concerned with the well-being of her charges, Jacobs worried for her daughter's and the other teachers' health.[141] Having been sick while working as the Willis family's nurse, Jacobs knew that health expertise would not inoculate against illness. Modeling the community concern for others' health for which she advocated, Jacobs wrote from Alexandria in 1864, "I find the exposure and hard work is wearing upon the teachers."[142] The following year, in a letter in the *Freedmen's Record*, Jacobs elaborated: "My daughter's health will not allow her to be confined to the school. She has charge of the Industrial Department, is teacher in the sabbath school, and assists me in my out-door work. We need another teacher."[143] New England Freedmen's Aid Society took her claim seriously. Later that year, a call for teacher applicants in the *Freedmen's Record* listed "health" as the first qualification for the job.[144] Like both her mother before her and Harper's Iola Leroy, whose "undermined" health ultimately makes her "quite unequal to the task" of teacher, Louisa's professional responsibility for the well-being of others ultimately compromises her own health.[145]

Jacobs understood this illness as a direct result of the devaluation of Black women's care labor. In an 1864 report to the New York Yearly Meeting of the Society of Friends, she writes, "Hard work is wearing sadly on the teachers. The doctor says my daughter will have to give up; but her heart is in the work. More teachers are needed, but we have no accommodations for them. The rations they give colored teachers amount to very little, and it would take every dollar of their pay to board them."[146] Louisa, Jacobs explains, is overworked. This passage echoes a sentiment that Jacobs conveyed to Amy Post at the height of her illness at Idlewild: "I can never get well while I am at a service."[147] But just as economic need drove Jacobs to labor while ill, limited funding meant that Jacobs could not employ enough staff to offset the demands on Louisa's limited energy. While white abolitionist accounts of Jacobs's relief work celebrated her for being "unwearied in her labors," Jacobs refused to romanticize the caregiver's body.

Illness and disability, Jacobs demonstrates, are not only consequences of enslavement and its aftermath; they can also be produced by the exhausting efforts to ameliorate such impairments. Both Stephen Knadler and Todd Carmody have examined how the "disciplinary" rhetoric of "rehabilitation" and "cure" became central to uplift ideology in the early twentieth century.

By highlighting the physical precarity of those who work to cultivate health, however, Jacobs reckons with how efforts toward "improvement" themselves can cause harm.[148] C. Riley Snorton has argued that Jacobs documents "performances *for* rather than *of* freedom" in *Incidents* by "imagining other qualities of life and being for those marked by and for captivity."[149] Her descriptions of caregiving operate within a similarly fugitive register, as Jacobs shows that health, like freedom, remains tentative. For Jacobs, the bodily freedom attained by emancipation does not necessarily facilitate a stable state of health or able-bodiedness, but rather initiates an ongoing negotiation of caregiving's demands.

A decade after Jacobs began establishing schools for formerly enslaved children, another type of educational institution emerged under the banner of "reform." The founding of the Carlisle Indian Industrial School in 1879 inaugurated a widespread movement of institutions that promised to "civilize" Indigenous children by instilling white Christian values—including those related to domestic health. While Jacobs worried about the working conditions that impaired women teachers' health in Black Reconstruction-era schools, the health of pupils—and especially young girls—was a crucial and contentious matter among educators at Carlisle. As I demonstrate in the next chapter, ideas about student health were essential both to white teachers' justification of their instructional methods and to Indigenous critiques of the schools' injurious practices.

CHAPTER FOUR

Pedagogies of Disability at the Carlisle Indian Industrial School

In May of 1896, the Carlisle Indian Industrial School's weekly newspaper, *The Indian Helper*, ran a brief anonymous entry criticizing Indigenous people's lack of health knowledge. "They do not know anything about physiology," the author claimed. "They know nothing about the laws of health. They do not understand the meaning of sanitation."[1] This apparently widespread crisis could be attributed, the article insisted, to "Ignorant Indian Mothers" who the author claimed were guided by their love for their children rather than by responsible observation of the "laws"—a term that neatly captured the role that governmental systems played in ideas about health. Indeed, the logic of the article justified the school's federally funded colonial project. If Indigenous women could not be trusted to care for their own children, then the off-reservation boarding school system could be understood as a public health intervention. The author in *The Indian Helper* vehemently insisted that Native mothers' ignorance has severe consequences; these declarations of Indigenous incompetence were printed under the headline: "Why Indian Children Die So Young."

The article's threatening, morbid title placed blame squarely on the shoulders of Native women while simultaneously obscuring the histories of colonial violence that actually caused widespread Indigenous death—including at Carlisle itself. Operated in Carlisle, Pennsylvania, the Carlisle Indian Industrial School was the first of a host of government-established and federally funded off-reservation boarding schools that separated Indigenous children from their families and nations with the aim of assimilating them to European American norms. Overseen by the Bureau of Indian Affairs, the school applied a militaristic approach to its pupils both in the rigid routines of daily life and in the construction of Indigenous cultures as enemy forces. The school's founder, military officer Richard Henry Pratt, frankly described his mission as "kill the Indian, save the man," and the educational movement he initiated often did the former. Historians have shown that tuberculosis and other infectious diseases were highly prevalent during the first few decades of off-reservation Indigenous education. While educators claimed that residential schools rescued Native children from the unhygienic homes for which they held mothers responsible, their own negligence encouraged the spread of disease and, in many cases, death. Students living in crowded conditions were forced to share inadequately sanitized resources such as linens and school supplies, and as many as three could be required to occupy a single bed.[2] In this chapter, I take up both the prevalence of settler educators' claims that assimilationist education could improve Native peoples' health and accounts of the physical debilitation that Indigenous students actually experienced at the hands of this curriculum.[3] While the previous two chapters examined how the labor of caring for others could be a strenuous and even injurious undertaking, this chapter considers the potential dangers posed to the presumed beneficiaries of physical education knowledge.

Exemplars of what Kyla Schuller refers to as "biophilanthropy," off-reservation boarding schools were driven by "the use of children as an instrument of settler colonialism."[4] As presumed arbiters of the home and school with the power to shape the bodies and minds of ensuing generations, Native girls were viewed as especially valuable tools in the project of "civilizing" Indigenous communities.[5] K. Tsianina Lomawaima (Mvskoke/Creek, not enrolled) explains that the "federal agenda . . . was to train Indian girls in subservience and submission," preparing them to "support[ ] their husbands in the difficult climb up the cultural evolutionary staircase."[6] Vocational programs enlisted female students as workers in settler homes as part of a curriculum that both exploited their physical labor and enacted a process of "erasure and replacement" with regard to Indigenous domestic and familial arrangements.[7]

The logic of Carlisle and the many boarding schools that emulated its pedagogy was predicated on what Liat Ben-Moshe calls the "racial criminal pathologization" of Native pupils.[8] In the era of muscular Christianity, moral and physical character were understood as mutually constitutive, and Native "savages" were accused of lacking both. Educators operated within what Jess L. Wilcox Cowing has termed a "settler ableist" framework that deemed Native children innately impaired and defined human value according to perceived able-bodiedness.[9] While, as I argued in chapter 1, Margaret Fuller's similar assessment of Indigenous girls' bodies in the early 1840s led her to imagine them as ineligible for physical education, late nineteenth-century educators were committed to rehabilitating what they perceived as their Native pupils' defects. When Pratt claimed that "the Indian could learn to march in line with America as a very part of it, head up, eyes front," he meant this quite literally.[10] The extensive physical education curriculum he developed included explicit exercise instruction along with disciplinary, vocational, and religious training that aimed to regulate the body as well as the mind and spirit in order to render students "fit" for "civilization."[11]

Educators' attempts to cultivate able-bodied, "civilized" pupils produced widespread debility, and students were attuned to their schooling's significant corporeal consequences.[12] Luther Standing Bear (Oglala Lakota), a member of Carlisle's first graduating class, recalled of his time at the school, "we had to get used to so many things we had never known before that it worked on our nerves to such an extent that it told on our bodies."[13] Rather than serve as the conduits of "civilization" educators hoped for, students' malleable bodies registered the trauma of their incarceration at the school. The social and discursive construction of Native youth as disabled and, according to settler ableist logic, in need of rehabilitation, ultimately led to their material impairment.[14] While the "social model" sometimes propagated within disability studies scholarship differentiates between "disability" as social exclusion and "impairment" as bodily condition, such a distinction breaks down when the material repercussions of social forces come into focus.[15] "Discourse," Sami Schalk and Jina B. Kim explain, "justifies and shores up structural power relations, leading to eventual material impact on marginalized people."[16] As a pedagogical science that translated constructed ideals into material expectations, physical education was a central mechanism through which settler ableist logic exerted itself on the bodies of Native youth.

I focus my analysis on the years 1897 to 1900, a period that saw both the appointment of a female superintendent of Indian schools, Estelle Reel, and the tenure of one of Carlisle's most famous teachers, the Yankton writer Zitkala-Ša.[17] I begin by illuminating the gendered notions of health and morality espoused by Reel and her fellow settler educators, who were convinced that their Indigenous pupils were physically inferior and thus in need of a curative education. From there, I turn to the autobiographical writings that Zitkala-Ša published in the *Atlantic Monthly* in 1900, a year after she taught music and oratory at Carlisle.[18] Penelope Kelsey (Seneca descent) argues that because assimilationist schools viewed a regulated body as a measure of mental and moral transformation, the embodied experiences of boarding school narrators constitute "unexamined sites of indigenous knowledge formation."[19] As such, I join Cowing in reading Zitkala-Ša's writing as testifying to "the debilitating effects of white, Christian assimilation on young Native women and girls," and I situate this as a crucial counternarrative to the political promise of physical education espoused by many settler feminists.[20] I argue that while settler educators like Reel insisted that their pedagogy corrected for deficiencies in their Indigenous pupils' bodies, Zitkala-Ša inverts Carlisle's rehabilitative logic to illuminate the school's harmful effects. I conclude by considering the alternative embodiments that Zitkala-Ša imagines might provide not only physical but also spiritual relief.

"The White [Wo]Man's Power to Repair the Body"

Control over students' bodies was folded into nearly every aspect of education at Carlisle and the various off-reservation boarding schools modeled after it. John Nicholas Choate's now famous "before and after" photographs of Carlisle pupils make clear that educators believed corporeal transformation signified successful assimilation.[21] From exercise instruction sessions to disciplinary and vocational training, boarding school authorities exerted biopolitical authority by positioning the Indigenous body as in urgent need of management. Susan Burch argues that "ableist rationales ultimately reinforce settler colonial aspirations and further actions," and, indeed, educators' intentions of "civilizing" Native students was inextricable from their insistence that they were physiologically inferior.[22]

Educators at Carlisle routinely asserted students' corporeal inferiority, but with the caveat that the defects they perceived could be eradicated if properly attended. What Sean Kicummah Teuton (Cherokee) describes as the "implicit disability model" of US policies toward Native people was reflected in boarding schools' overwhelming emphasis on rehabilitating students' supposedly defective bodies.[23] Physical education was integral to this corrective effort from the start. In 1896, Indian school superintendent William Nicholas Hailmann recommended "persistent and systematic physical training in suitable games and methodical calisthenics and gymnastic exercises, in order to overcome the lack of grace and vigor in the general bearing and in the movements of the children."[24] The following year, the school's annual report announced proudly that "physical training indoors and out for both boys and girls continues to form a part of the regular daily routine of the school life."[25] These exercises were part of a broader disciplinary regime that extended beyond the gymnasium. In fact, sex-segregated physical education classes at Carlisle were supervised by the school's designated "disciplinarian," William Grant Thompson, a graduate of the Chautauqua Normal School of Physical Education.[26]

This link between discipline and health at Carlisle was clearly a product of Pratt's military background. He derived his methods primarily from his 1875 to 1878 experience as a military captain supervising a group of Indigenous

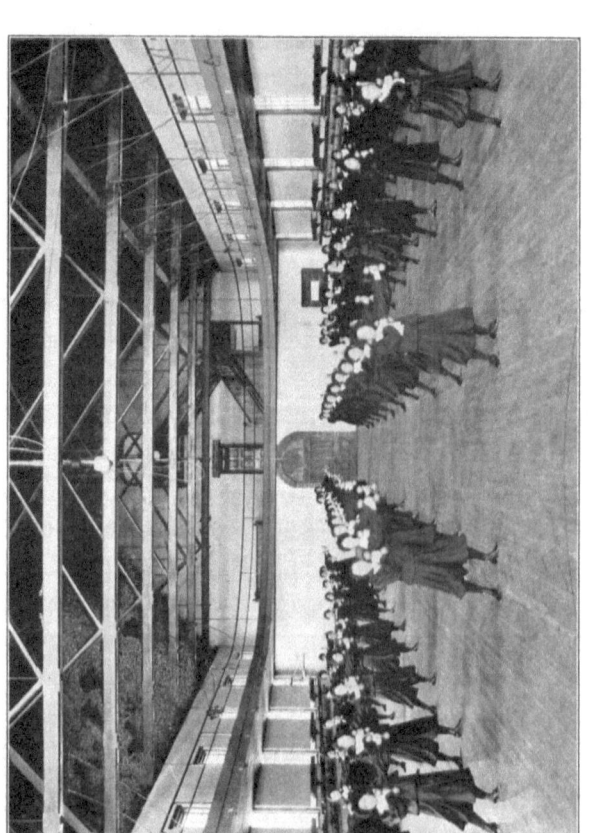

Photograph by Frances Benjamin Johnston of a girls' physical education class in the Carlisle gymnasium. Printed in the catalogue of the Indian Industrial School, 1902. Courtesy of Carlisle Indian School Digital Resource Center.

prisoners at Fort Marion, Florida, where he established an informal assimilationist educational program.[27] In his aptly titled memoir, *Battlefield and Classroom*, Pratt reveals the overlapping practices and ideologies that structured his treatment of military prisoners and pupils alike. Pratt explains that in addition to lessons in reading and writing English, those incarcerated at Fort Marion participated in "daily drills" of the military "setting up process" as well as "gymnastic exercises" that laid the groundwork for Carlisle's physical education program. Pratt insists that the prisoners at Fort Marion eventually developed an "interest in the white man's power to repair the body," which he claims "led the Indians to a greater desire to know and become part of our civilization."[28] This belief that a strengthened body could alter Native pupils' attitudes became central to the educational theories at Carlisle, where the Indigenous body was treated as both an object and an instrument of assimilation.

Upon its founding in 1879, the school's militaristic curriculum brought with it deeply entrenched ideas about American masculinity that were encapsulated by the concurrent popularity of war hero turned politician Theodore Roosevelt. Hayes Peter Mauro suggests that Roosevelt's rise provides important context for the military-influenced ideologies that governed off-reservation boarding schools. What Roosevelt famously referred to as "the strenuous life" provided a powerful model for educators' efforts to cultivate the physical and moral character they deemed prerequisite to national belonging.[29] Roosevelt represented a distinctly American strain of what was called "muscular Christianity." After originating in England in the mid-nineteenth century, muscular Christianity made its way to the United States largely through the establishment of the Young Men's Christian Association (YMCA) branches across the country that Roosevelt claimed in 1900 would "make men self-helpful" by teaching them to "not only be good, but strong."[30] Carlisle students founded one such branch on campus in the 1880s. Educators, too, presumed that the cultivation of such physical strength would beget the moral righteousness of what Roosevelt called "the true Christian" and "the true citizen" on whom a European American notion of civilization was premised.[31]

Roosevelt, who would become president three years later, appears in an 1898 issue of *The Indian Helper* as a paragon of responsible, healthy, European American habits. The anonymous author critiques students' refusal to wear warm garments in inclement weather by framing this behavior as violating the conduct Roosevelt modeled. The article explains that while "others got sick and died" during the Spanish-American War, Roosevelt "was not sick a day"—he "understands the laws of hygiene," which he observed because "he knew that he could do his best work for his country if he had a strong, well body."[32] The anonymous author then encourages all pupils to be like the "Roosevelt boys and girls who do not neglect the essentials to good health."[33]

Importantly, these "Roosevelt boys and girls" were presented not as a monolith, but as two separate populations with distinct relationships to health. The author describes the ideal students as boys who "put on overshoes when they are obliged to go out in slush and snow" and "girls who . . . put on their wraps in going from sewing room, dining-hall and laundry to quarters."[34] By dressing warmly in cold weather, the entry suggests, students "will grow up to be strong men and women, ready for football, or for the sturdy avocations of life that require sound bodies and minds."[35] Health, according to this logic, requires compliance with the school's sex-specific health norms: sports for boys and domestic labor for girls. Such gendered health advice was a common feature of *The Indian Helper*. "Do you want to be graceful?" asks an 1888 piece with the instructive title "Girls Read This." "If you do," the entry continues, "practice this movement: Stand squarely on the soles of the feet then raise and lower the body upon the ball of the feet and toes, making the movements repeatedly for several minutes. This will help you to walk easily and lightly, never walk heavily on the heel, throw weight of the body on the ball of the foot if you wish to walk well."[36] Such instruction solidified able-bodiedness as integral to the image of "civilized" Native youth that Carlisle promoted, and it figured "civilized" femininity as an "eas[y]" "light[ness]" that paradoxically required effortful "practice."

The publication that offered this advice, *The Indian Helper*, was printed and composed by students under the guidance of Superintendent of Printing Marianna Burgess. As Amelia V. Katanski argues, the newspaper functioned as "a rhetorical panopticon that encouraged student self-colonization through writing."[37] Burgess, who consistently worked to influence student self-perception, did so most famously by penning *Stiya: A Carlisle Indian Girl at Home*, a fictionalized 1891 narrative for which she appropriated the persona of Carlisle student, Stiya Kowacura, and used the image of another, Lucy Tsisnah, for the author photo.[38] Burgess's penchant for publishing health content could be similarly distorting. In addition to the narrow model of femininity she promoted in articles such as "Girls Read This," she also reprinted health texts with deceptive framing. Echoing the false authorship of *Stiya*, Burgess published a short poem in 1886 entitled "A Fourteen Year Old Girl's Good Advice." The poem consists of a set of health maxims including "take the open air," "freely exercise," "eat the simplest food," and "drink the pure cold water," and the title suggests that these are the recommendations of a young woman, presumably a student at the school.[39] In reality, though, the rhyme, which dates to at least 1855 and was often put to music, was originally titled "Sense-Opathy." By implying that this European American advice was penned by a young Native student, Burgess creates a fictionalized model of the thoroughly assimilated Indian girl, and she reveals how central domestic health knowledge was to this ideal.

Intersecting ideas about health and gender became further entrenched in the curriculum of assimilationist education after the 1898 appointment of Estelle Reel as superintendent of Indian schools. Shortly after assuming her post, Reel traveled across the country visiting boarding schools and training faculty. Reel codified her pedagogical recommendations in her instruction manual for educators, *Course of Study for the Indian Schools of the United States. Industrial and Literary* (1901), a document that historian Lomawaima has called "a blueprint for total control of people—mental, physical, and moral."[40] Reel practiced a kind of "settler feminism" insofar as she gained her own political power and authority through the imposition of patriarchal norms on Indigenous women.[41] When it came to the education of Indigenous girls specifically, Reel focused primarily on domestic science. At Carlisle and the schools modeled after it, female pupils were largely responsible for cleaning, cooking, and laundry. Though possibly a product of the schools' limited budget, this use of student labor was also coded as valuable instruction.[42] Reel writes in her *Course* that "the ideal training for girls is that which will instill a love for home and make good, neat housekeepers."[43]

These lessons had distinctly colonial aims. Reel writes, "the art of housekeeping . . . is what we want to teach our Indian girls, assuring them that because our grandmothers did things in a certain way is no reason why we should do the same."[44] Reel's call for students to reject their "grandmothers'" ways of living, like the disparaging of "Ignorant Indian Mothers" in *The Indian Helper*, reflects Mary Zaborskis's formulation of assimilation education as a process of "orphaning" that left Native children unable either "to carry on Indianness through the Native body" or to "leave behind their Native bodies in the eyes of the state."[45] When Reel explains that "the good housekeeper is the arbiter of the health of the occupants of the home," she does not simply echo the tenets of eighteenth-century republican motherhood, but rather inverts the earlier infantilizing of racialized domestic workers discussed in chapter 2 to imagine Indigenous girls as maternal figures in white homes.[46] Indeed, they trained students for precisely such roles. Carlisle students were often sent to live with and work for European American families as part of the school's

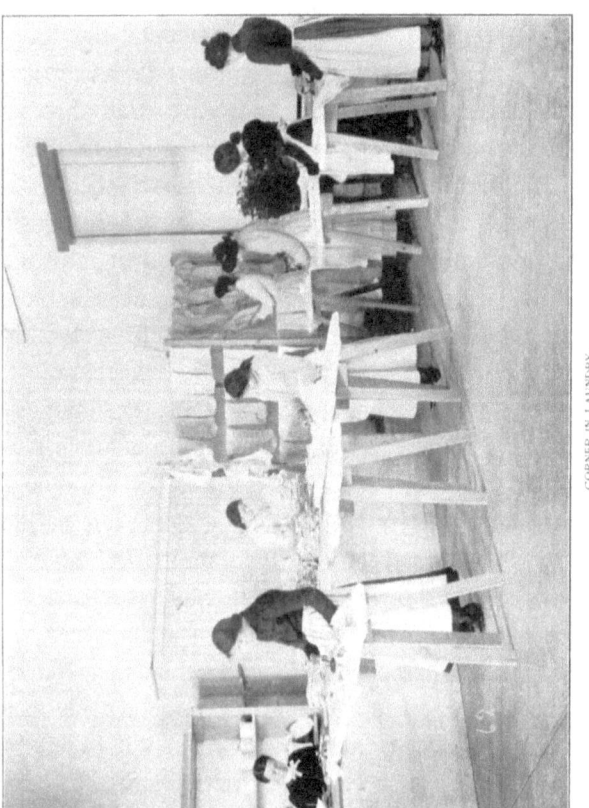

Photograph by Frances Benjamin Johnston of girls laundering at Carlisle. Printed in the catalogue of the Indian Industrial School, 1902. Courtesy of Carlisle Indian School Digital Resource Center.

"outing program." Pratt explicitly modeled this program after American chattel slavery. He believed that "through forcing Negroes to live among us and become producers, slavery became a more humane and real civilizer, Americanizer, and promoter of usefulness for the Negro," and he was convinced that "this lesson . . . in some way should be applied to the Indian."[47] Reel thoroughly endorsed the program and recommended it be adopted at other off-reservation boarding schools as well, since "association with good white people is the best civilizing agency that can be devised."[48]

Given that Carlisle equated civilization with health, it is no surprise that one educator remarked that upon returning from their "outings," girls were "almost invariably in better health than when they went out; they are usually fleshier, with clearer, better complexions," and, as a result, "they have quite the appearance of a party of white girls."[49] Such assimilationist "improvements" were seen as a product of their domestic education. As a result of the program, Reel explained, "the girl . . . is trained in the practical everyday life of the household; gains the ability to cook, to sew, and to wash; forms those habits of cleanliness and order so necessary to a comfortable home; and becomes in every respect a thorough housewife."[50] Educators hoped that this immersive—and exploitative—experience would not only train students in settler domestic science, but also teach them to see the value of these practices. At the 1900 meeting of the National Education Association's Department of Indian Education, Josephine E. Richards, a teacher at the Hampton Normal and Industrial Institute, insisted that the "outing system" that originated at Carlisle had the benefit of "fostering a 'noble discontent' with the dirt and disorder" that Richards and many in her audience associated with traditional Native homes.[51]

Such preparation for housekeeping was framed as a form of scientific training. Outlining the importance of Indigenous girls' domestic education at the 1900 National Education Association (NEA) meeting, Richards implored attendees to "consider some of the crying needs of the Indian home of the present day, and also the training which will best fit the Indian girls in our schools to meet those needs."[52] She claimed it was urgent that these girls learn not only the art of homemaking, but also the science. If they were expected to manage orderly, hygienic homes as adults, she explained, these students would need either "a text-book on physiology and hygiene" or "simple oral lessons . . . along these lines."[53] In order to "become the true uplifter of the home" in the fashion of middle-class European American women, she suggested, Native girls would need to be versed in the human body and its management.

Domestic instruction was also presented as explicitly health-promoting. In her *Course*, Reel declares it the institution's responsibility to provide pupils with an education that will "counteract the influences of unfortunate heredity and strengthen the physique."[54] Indeed, she writes that because "the Indian child is of lower physical organization than the white child," such pupils "cannot be taught like the children of the white man until they are taught to do like them."[55] For Reel, the transformation of the students' bodies was thus an essential first step in instilling the norms of a "civilization" that was profoundly shaped by gender. A 1900 entry in *The Indian Helper* on "The Exercise That Makes Healthy Girls" reflected this attitude, insisting that "to keep the complexion and spirits good, to preserve grace, strength, and agility of motion, there is no gymnasium so valuable, no exercise more beneficial in results than sweeping, dusting, making beds, washing dishes and polishing of brass and silver."[56] While the Carlisle gymnasium was a source of immense pride for the school, the author of this piece suggests that "it is more healthful to complete chores than to perform the drills . . . with Indian clubs, dumb-bells, etc., practicing different movements, in perfect time to music" that were a common sight in the gymnasium.[57] By framing household chores as exercise itself, the author recalls a much earlier model of women's physical education. Nearly sixty years after Catharine Beecher proposed that "performing domestic duties" provided women with "triple benefit" compared to "long and formal walks, merely for exercise," this gendered Victorian notion reemerges to suggest that, for Indigenous girls, domestic labor itself was construed as an ideal form of physical education.[58]

An Injurious Education

By the time she arrived at Carlisle in 1897 to teach music and oratory, Zitkala-Ša was already well acquainted with the forms of physical education the school promoted. As a student at White's Manual Labor Institute in Indiana years prior, Zitkala-Ša had been required to participate in standard exercises such as "club swinging and field drill, for the purpose of aiding physical development."[59] There, she was also responsible for an array of domestic tasks, including "sewing, care of dining-room, dish-washing, cooking, baking, care of milk, laundrying, and chamber-work."[60] Both of these forms physical education, as well as the institution's strict code of conduct, emerge in the pages of her 1900 short story, "The School Days of an Indian Girl." Written the year after she left her teaching position at Carlisle, the story ostensibly recalls her childhood education at White's, but it also inevitably invokes the culture of her former workplace.

Throughout the story, she shows how bodily regimentation was woven into the fabric of daily life at the school. Immediately upon her arrival at the institution depicted in "School Days," Zitkala-Ša and her companions are "placed in a line of girls who were marching into the dining room."[61] Becoming a pupil of the institution, the story makes clear early on, requires her to quite literally fall into step with her peers. The rules she describes as "needlessly binding" were physically as well as psychologically confining, and students' movements were scripted throughout the day.[62] During her first dinner at the school, Zitkala-Ša finds that even meals are thoroughly choreographed:

> A small bell was tapped, and each of the pupils drew a chair from under the table. Supposing this act meant they were to be seated, I pulled out mine and at once slipped into it from one side. But when I turned my head, I saw that I was the only one seated, and all the rest at our table remained standing. Just as I began to rise, looking shyly around to see how chairs were to be used, a second bell was sounded. All were seated at last, and I had to crawl back into my chair again. I heard a man's voice at one end of the hall, and I looked around to see him. But all the others hung their heads over their plates. As I glanced at the long chain of tables, I caught the eyes of a paleface woman upon me.[63]

The scene unfolds as a series of asynchronous movements. Zitkala-Ša sits when others stand, rises when they are seated, and seems always to be looking in the wrong direction. The other students' coordinated comportment—what she calls "eating by formula"—as well as the teacher's chastising gaze suggest that mastering such routine actions will be an important part of her training at the schools.[64]

Zitkala-Ša further illustrates the institution's quotidian disciplining of students' bodies through her depictions of dress. Upon their arrival, students at off-reservation boarding schools were dressed in European American uniforms, and the impact of this required transformation permeates Zitkala-Ša's accounts. As the famous "before and after" photographs of Carlisle students' wardrobe changes make clear, educators quite literally stripped Native youth of their tribal identities to argue that they had been successfully "civilized." While, as C. Daniel Redmond argues, Zitkala-Ša was attuned to clothing's rhetorical power in her public appearances, her stories are less concerned with what clothing signifies visually than with how it dictates the movements of the body it adorns.[65] Zitkala-Ša's attention to clothing's kinetic effects begins in her story about life on the Yankton Reservation, "Impressions of an Indian Childhood" (1900). There, she describes her childhood wardrobe: "loosely clad in a slip of brown buckskin, and light-footed with a pair of soft moccasins on my feet, I was as free as the wind that blew my hair."[66] Her freedom of movement here is explicitly facilitated by the pliable garments she will soon be prohibited from wearing. The "heavy blanket" she dons for her journey to the school similarly makes her "happy" during her walk with her mother to the carriage.[67] Upon her arrival, however, the comforting material is taken away, as is her control over her bodily movements. "I felt like sinking to the floor," she recalls, "for my blanket had been stripped from my shoulders."[68] The removal of traditional clothing here constitutes not only a symbolic loss, but a visceral, embodied sensation. The physical transformation produced by this wardrobe change is further underscored by her observation of the "Indian girls" wearing "stiff shoes and closely clinging dresses."[69] She is stunned by their comportment as they march in their "tightly fitting clothes," stripped of the freedom of mobility offered by her "loose" buckskin dress and blanket.[70]

Zitkala-Ša illustrates, too, the school's use of students' disciplined bodies as a source of domestic labor. She recalls being "sent into the kitchen to mash the turnips for dinner," a food she found "offensive."[71] She begins by performing the expected actions—"I stood upon a step, and, grasping the handle with both hands"—before transforming the labor into an outlet for her "hot rage" and "work[ing] [her] vengeance upon" the vegetables.[72] Parodying the health benefits Reel and others insisted such chores could provide, Zitkala-Ša reports that her "energy was renewed" by the task.[73] She writes, "I felt a satisfying sensation that the weight of my body had gone into it," though "it" here is not a delight in domestic productivity but a sense of having rebelled against the constraints of the school's curriculum.[74]

Another much-cited section of "School Days" titled "Iron Routine" further describes the extent to which students' movements were regulated by school administrators. Zitkala-Ša recalls being woken early in the morning "from happy dreams of Western rolling lands and unlassoed freedom," forced to relinquish the freedom of movement described in "Impressions."[75] "We had a short time," she recalls, "to jump into our shoes and clothes, and wet our eyes with icy water, before a small hand bell was vigorously rung for roll call," at which point "we rushed downstairs, bounding over two high steps at a time, to land in the assembly room."[76] The strict choreography of the daily roll call appears here a form of exercise, as students "jump" and "bound" into place. Signs of disability and illness, however, complicate this scene of athleticism. She writes of teachers taking attendance, "no matter if a dull headache or the painful cough of slow consumption had delayed the absentee, there was only time enough to mark the tardiness."[77] By coding the daily morning routine as a form of physical education, Zitkala-Ša reveals how supposedly rehabilitative practices could actually cause and exacerbate students' impairments.

Zitkala-Ša makes clear that the curriculum educators claimed would develop pupils' bodies could also have the opposite effect. Of her education, she writes, "I have many times trudged in the day's harness heavy-footed, like a dumb sick brute."[78] Her description of the curriculum as "the day's harness" also reveals her identity as a laborer within an educational system that exploited her body both on campus and in European American families' homes as part of the "outing program." The imposition of that harness also signals that she is not innately impaired or "brut[ish]," but is made that way by school's rigid expectations and exhausting expectations. Zitkala-Ša's description of the physical effects of the demands of boarding school labor reveal how physical training exploited students' bodies as potentially productive labor sources, often devastating and debilitating them in the process.[79]

Indeed, Zitkala-Ša's health worsens over the course of her time at the school.[80] The process of her debilitation begins onboard the train headed east in "School Days" when she observes "the lonely figure of my mother vanish[ing] in the distance" and becomes "suddenly weak, as if I might fall limp to the ground."[81] This sudden sense of "weakness" persists throughout the story, in which her new environment leaves her "trembling."[82] She documents the death of a classmate, too, who, rather than "bound" into place as was expected of her, "used to mope along at my side, until one morning she could not raise her head from her pillow."[83] The young Zitkala-Ša blames her friend's death on "the paleface woman," whom she accuses of "cruel neglect of our physical ills."[84] Far from developing students' bodies, she suggests, educators are directly responsible for their deterioration. "Like a slender tree," she writes of her education in another 1900 story, "An Indian Teacher among Indians," "I had been uprooted from my mother, nature, and God. I was shorn of my branches, which had waved in sympathy and love for home and friends. The natural coat of bark which had protected my oversensitive nature was scraped off to the very quick."[85] Her own and other Indigenous youths' schooling, she suggests, is indeed a physical transformation, one that Cowing notes Zitkala-Ša likens to settler deforestation.[86] The curriculum is not, however, a process of physical growth, as settler educators insisted, but rather a systematic method of physical debilitation.

When she eventually becomes a teacher at Carlisle, Zitkala-Ša, who experienced fatigue, lung infection, and stomach illness throughout her adult life, is in the throes of illness. She describes arriving at the school "frail and languid," with "exhausted strength."[87] Recalling her first "sultry month" on campus, she is struck by the "recklessness" of her having remained in that stifling environment despite "nature's warning."[88] "Fortunately," she adds, "my inheritance of a marvelous endurance enabled me to bend without breaking."[89] Here she counters the beliefs espoused by Pratt and Reel that Native children were physiologically inferior and in need of rehabilitation by suggesting that an "inherit[ed]" capacity to "endur[e]" is what enables her to survive *despite* the school's interventions.

She makes a similar case elsewhere in the essay when describing visitors to Carlisle: "From morning till evening, many specimens of civilized peoples visited the Indian school. The city folks with canes and eyeglasses, the countrymen with sunburnt cheeks and clumsy feet, forgot their relative social ranks in an ignorant curiosity. Both sorts of these Christian palefaces were alike astounded at seeing the children of savage warriors so docile and industrious."[90] Such visits were common practice at Carlisle. In Pratt's view, Carlisle's "public presentation of its students" effectively "served as the department of publicity in Indian school work," and students regularly performed military drills and participated in athletic games for audiences not only at on-campus events such as graduation, but also at various fairs and festivals.[91] Zitkala-Ša's ironic account turns the evaluative gaze back on the spectators to assess these "specimens" physically. What unites the "city folks" and "country men" are the mobility impairments signified by their "canes" and "clumsy feet." The students, in contrast, exhibit what the viewers would consider bodily mastery, underscoring the hypocrisy of constructing Indigenous youth as uniquely impaired and thus in need of civilizing.

Having established Native students' potential for vitality, Zitkala-Ša explicitly frames her own illness as a product of her education when she writes of her mother, "had she known of my worn condition, she would have said the white man's papers were not worth the freedom and health I had lost by them."[92] In fact, upon meeting Pratt, who appears in "An Indian Teacher" as her "stately gray-haired . . . employer," Zitkala-Ša immediately experiences "a leaden weakness . . . as if years of weariness lay like water-soaked logs upon me."[93] Pratt himself emerges here as an embodiment of the school's injurious force as his physical presence incites the "weariness" produced by her subjection to a curriculum of his design.

Zitkala-Ša further illustrates how European American approaches to physical education could produce bodily harm in her 1902 essay, "A Protest against the Abolition of the Indian Dance." Though it appeared after her departure from the institution, she published the essay in the Carlisle school newspaper, which had by then been renamed the *Red Man and Helper*. Eleven years before she coauthored *The Sun Dance Opera*, which celebrated embodied Indigenous spiritual practices and featured Ute dancers in its live performances, Zitkala-Ša's essay points out the hypocrisy of efforts to ban Native dances. As a counterexample, she describes a scene of "whirling couples in pretty rhythm to orchestral music," but reminds readers that the women's "fair bodies are painfully corseted" in "steel frames" and sardonically cites this injurious dance practice as evidence of the enduring influence of "the barbaric Teutons and Anglo-Saxons."[94] Coding European Americans' ancestry as "barbaric," she exposes the arbitrariness of references to Native "savages" and proposes that so-called "civilized" forms of dance and bodily expression pose an immediate threat to women's health.

Later in the essay, however, Zitkala-Ša questions the notion that "any graceful movement of the human figure in rhythm to music was ever barbaric" by turning to the purported health benefits of dance.[95] "Scientists," she explains, "advise an occasional relaxation of work or daily routine with such ardor that even the inmates of the insane asylums are allowed to dance their dances."[96] Here dance is not simply recreational but also therapeutic. The implied health benefits of such activity mirror Reel's and others' claims that physical education could be rehabilitative. Zitkala-Ša's reference to "inmates of insane asylums" is also significant. The Canton Asylum, a psychiatric facility that exclusively detained Indigenous people, was established near the Yankton Reservation in South Dakota in 1902, the same year Zitkala-Ša published this essay.[97] Though she doesn't refer to Canton itself, Zitkala-Ša does highlight the shared disenfranchisement of Indigenous and disabled people, concluding the essay by arguing that "if it is right for the insane and idiot to dance, the Indian (who is classified with them) should have the same privilege."[98] Through the language of classification and "privilege," she clearly alludes to the denial of both groups' rights. Publishing the essay in the Carlisle school newspaper, however, she also invokes what Ben-Moshe calls the parallel "carceral locales" of the asylum and the Indian school, both of which were premised on the supposed biological inferiority of residents.[99] Though institutionalized, she observes of the asylum "inmates" that they are "allowed to dance *their* dances." Therapeutic movement, she therefore suggests, should be extended to Indigenous pupils not by teaching the standardized comportments that Carlisle educators demanded, but by allowing communities to perform their own forms of bodily expression.[100]

Alternative Embodiments

Zitkala-Ša's framing of her own debilitation as akin to that of a "slender tree" that has been "uprooted," "shorn of . . . branches" and "scraped" of "bark" alludes to both bodily harm and Yankton beliefs regarding well-being. "For the white man's papers," she writes of her education, "I had given up my faith in the Great Spirit. For these same papers I had forgotten the healing in trees and brooks."[101] If "trees," as she suggests here, are a "healing" force parallel to that of "the Great Spirit," whom educators have tried to supplant with Christianity, then her depiction of her own impairments as the mutilation of a tree illuminates the intertwinement of spiritual and physical health. Her reunion with her mother further establishes this connection. When her mother tells her, "I have been praying steadfastly to the Great Spirit to avenge our wrongs," Zitkala-Ša deems this effort futile, as her own "shattered energy" has left her "unable to hold longer any faith."[102] Her physical impairment, she suggests here, directly impedes her spirituality. Though she would later convert to Catholicism, Zitkala-Ša fiercely resisted Christian indoctrination in her 1902 essay, "Why I Am a Pagan." Throughout the piece, she revises the emphasis on physicality espoused by the Carlisle YMCA and other proponents of muscular Christianity. While she had suggested two years earlier in "An Indian Teacher" that illness impedes spirituality, "Why I Am a Pagan" depicts a series of embodied practices that facilitate spirituality while also accommodating the physical fatigue she experienced.

"Why I Am a Pagan" elaborates on the "spirit" Zitkala-Ša introduces in "Impressions" and then reports having "lost" in her later stories. In "Impressions," she writes of her childhood freedom of movement, "It was as if . . . my hands and feet were only experiments for my spirit to work upon."[103] "Why I Am a Pagan" examines that "working" more closely by providing a detailed description of a religious experience. From the opening lines of the essay, she situates spirituality in the body. "When the spirit swells my breast," she begins, "I love to roam leisurely among the green hills; or sometimes, sitting on the brink of the murmuring Missouri, I marvel at the great blue overhead."[104] A far cry from the robust physicality of muscular Christianity, this "leisurely" ambulation is followed by moments of stillness that further denote her departure from a religious ethos of vigorous activity. "During the idle while I sat upon the sunny river brink," she reflects, "I grew somewhat," suggesting the transformative power of corporeal passivity.[105] Her contemplation of nature culminates in observations of the "Yellow Breast" bird, in whom she recognizes a model of spirituality. "Truly does it seem," she writes of the bird, "his vigorous freedom lies more in his little spirit than in his wing," minimizing the corporeal in favor of a more intangible source of vitality.[106]

The site of this embodied experience further politicizes Zitkala-Ša's actions. The transformative physical activity described in "Why I Am a Pagan" doesn't only counter settler physical education's insistence on rigid, regimented exercises. It also offers an ecological model of health that Cowing refers to as the "narrative link between land, health, and identity" in Zitkala-Ša's boarding school stories.[107] If, as Siobhan Senier puts it, "the mutual constitution of Indigeneity and disability is fundamentally about land expropriation," then Zitkala-Ša's purposeful interpolation into the landscape she describes constitutes a form of healing that refutes the colonial health models premised on Native displacement described in chapter 1.[108]

These illustrations of embodied and emplaced spiritual reverie unsettle a binary view of the Indigenous body as either ideal and uncolonized or sickened by colonialism. As Teuton explains, "the Indigenous body is too often either a romanticized and pristine pre-contact Native body to be revered, or a gritty, broken, tainted, even monstrous body to be feared or pitied," and these absolute characterizations remain "fixed at the poles of ability and disability."[109] Indeed, the contrast between the unencumbered "wild little girl" Zitkala-Ša compares to a "bounding deer" in "Impressions" and the debilitated condition she describes at the beginning of "An Indian Teacher" seem to uphold this paradigm.[110] "Why I Am a Pagan," however, steps outside this framework by presenting an embodied practice rooted in land and Yankton spirituality that "declares and resists disabling colonialism . . . but also acknowledges the spectrum of human variation and its limits on human ability."[111] That is, Zitkala-Ša rejects Pratt's "perfectible" Indigenous physique in favor of what Teuton calls a "sustainable" model of disability that is deeply connected to the environment.[112]

This entwinement of embodiment with "spirit" culminates in a direct confrontation between Yankton and Christian religious ideology when Zitkala-Ša describes conversing with a "native preacher" who laments her refusal to convert. At the end of their encounter, when "the church bell rang," he immediately "hurried forth," not unlike the students impelled to action by the "loud-clamoring bell" in "School Days."[113] "I watched him as he hastened along," she recalls of the preacher, "his eyes bent fast upon the dusty road till he disappeared at the end of a quarter of a mile."[114] With his hasty movement and downcast eyes, the preacher is wholly oblivious to the natural landscape that provides Zitkala-Ša with spiritual fulfillment earlier in the essay.

She concludes "Why I Am a Pagan" by extending this religious confrontation to the scene of writing itself. She explains that "the little incident" with the preacher "recalled to mind the copy of a missionary paper brought to my notice a few days ago, in which a 'Christian' pugilist commented upon a recent article of mine, grossly perverting the spirit of my pen."[115] Here she likely refers to Pratt, who published a scathing critique of her work in the April 1901 issue of the *Red Man and Helper*:

> All that Zitkalasa [sic] has in the way of literary ability and culture she owes to the good people, who, from time to time have taken her into their homes and hearts and given her aid. Yet not a word of gratitude or allusion to such kindness on the part of her friends has ever escaped her in any line of anything she has written for the public. By this course she injures herself and harms the educational work in progress for the race from which she sprang. In a list of educated Indians . . . we know no other case of such pronounced morbidness.[116]

Pratt, it seems, is what Zitkala-Ša calls a "'Christian' pugilist," or boxer, not only because of his commitment to a muscular model of Christian morality, but also due to his highly combative assertions of its supremacy over other forms of spirituality. Zitkala-Ša, who composed "Why I Am a Pagan" largely in response to Pratt, was apparently only briefly upset by his words. She reflects on his public criticism in a private 1901 letter, adopting Pratt's health-coded language to describe the impact of his words. "I feel sick way in my heart," she confesses. "I will recover from this nausea caused by the would be critics of my art. But I am ill at this moment."[117] Here as elsewhere, Zitkala-Ša presents Pratt and his assimilationist agenda as the source of her impairment. She does not "injure[] herself" or "harm the educational work," as Pratt suggests in the *Red Man and Helper*, but is rather sickened by it.

However, the letter takes a sudden, surprising, turn. "Ah — I rise. I lift my head!" she writes. "I laugh at the babble! I dare — I do! I guess I am not so sick after all."[118] Here Zitkala-Ša seemingly offers what Kelsey describes as "indigenous resistance . . . couched within an overcoming narrative" of disability.[119] The image of her triumphantly "lift[ing] her head" both recalls Pratt's idealized students "march[ing] in line with America . . . head up, eyes front," and contrasts that of her dying classmate who "could not raise her head from her pillow."[120] However, Zitkala-Ša's self-narration straddles these contradictory images of compliant and devastated students' bodies. Zitkala-Ša emerges from Pratt's criticism, as she does from his pedagogical authority, not as the vigorous, assimilated, and assimilating teacher he sought, but only as "not so sick." What she ultimately "dares" to do is not some Roosevelt-esque feat; instead, she responds to Pratt with "Why I Am a Pagan," in which idleness emerges as a form of embodied critique, a refusal of the "day's harness" and the productivity and degradation it implies. For Zitkala-Ša, the twin physical and spiritual threats of assimilationist education lie in the performances it demands of Indigenous students and teachers. Survival, she ultimately suggests, requires an alternative choreography.

Indigenous youth were not the only population to experience physical education as an instrument of assimilation. The "civilizing" model at Carlisle and similar schools was applied to less abuse ends in a growing settlement movement through which US-born white women across the country sought to instill "Americanness" in the children of European immigrants. As the next chapter demonstrates, definitions of what exactly constituted this American identity ranged widely from a romanticized notion of heterogeneous cosmopolitanism to a pursuit of homogeneous "fitness" influenced by the burgeoning eugenics movement.

CHAPTER FIVE

"Education for Citizenship" and the Immigrant Body

As the opening line of the 1896 manual, *School Gymnastics, Free Hand: A System of Physical Exercises for Schools* reveals, by the late nineteenth century, physical education advocacy was no longer the radical stance it had once been. "The advisability of including physical training in the school curriculum," the author, Jessie Hubbell Bancroft, writes, "is now so generally recognized that no plea seems necessary for its introduction."[1] Administrators and educators were by then well aware of their responsibility for pupils' physical as well as mental well-being. And yet problems persisted as instructors struggled to adapt methods derived from Europe to a US context. Bancroft quotes gymnastics instructor Baron Posse, writing that "Swedish gymnastics are good in Sweden for the Swedes, and German gymnastics in Germany for the Germans; but in America we are a conglomerate people, with different climate and conditions to deal with."[2] The American school itself, Bancroft insists, undermines physical education by limiting the period of daily exercise to a mere fifteen minutes and failing to provide adequate facilities. Swedish and German gymnastics have little value in the "restricted conditions . . . of the schoolroom," and so Bancroft offers a set of exercises tailored to the American context.[3]

Bancroft's introduction reflects two crucial developments at the turn of the twentieth century. First, she signals the growth of American physical education into an established field. Unlike her predecessors, she does not need to justify its place in school curricula, and she is strategic about how best to translate European methods into an emergent American model. A cofounder of the American Association for the Advancement of Physical Education and the future assistant director of physical education for the schools of Greater New York City, Bancroft represented a new class of women physical educators. Departing from its roots in domestic science, the late 1880s marked a turning point for the field.[4] No longer simply one aspect of a mother's or teacher's responsibilities, physical education became defined by professional, scientific expertise. Across the country, colleges and "normal schools" helmed largely by men with medical degrees began to prepare future gym teachers through rigorous and standardized training. Bancroft was a graduate of the Minneapolis

School of Physical Education, and later spent summers studying under leading expert Dudley Allen Sargent at Harvard's Hemenway Gymnasium.[5] In the decades that followed, a generation of women earned similar credentials at physical education normal schools across the country.

In addition to demonstrating the growing status of US physical education as a unique scientific discipline, Bancroft's introduction to *School Gymnastics* reflects the heterogeneity of the population that the field studied and trained. In the late nineteenth century, the United States was becoming, as Bancroft puts it, an increasingly "conglomerate" nation. Rates of immigration to the country exploded, and, as a result, foreign-born and first-generation American children represented an increasingly large portion of students receiving physical education instruction. As eugenics and other theories of physiological difference put immigrants' racialized bodies under intense scientific scrutiny, physical educators were forced to account for perceived physical differences in their pupils. How would they develop a physical education system that was distinct to the United States while also grappling with the nation's increasingly diverse population?

The wide range of possible answers to this problem is illustrated by the approaches to physical education articulated by Jane Addams and Charlotte Perkins Gilman. Though not professional physical educators themselves, both Addams and Gilman were invested in scientific approaches to child-rearing and adolescent development.[6] Both women insisted on the importance of specially trained expertise in the cultures they created—Addams at the Hull-House social settlement she founded in 1889, and Gilman in her utopian fiction of the 1910s. Two of the most prominent social reformers of the late nineteenth and early twentieth centuries, Addams and Gilman both were born in 1860 and died in 1935. The two remained friends and collaborators throughout their lives, joining forces on endeavors including the feminist publication *The Woman's Journal*, the Woman's Peace Party, and the American Sociological Society.[7] As waves of immigration rolled in from Southern and Eastern Europe, both Addams and Gilman positioned physical education as an important resource for these newcomers and their children.

The two women diverged, however, in their responses to the cultural and biological variance they perceived in these populations. Though the robust education programs Addams installed at Hull-House clearly influenced Gilman's thinking, the two differed significantly in their approaches to difference. Addams embraced the cultural diversity of her immigrant neighbors, insisting that the ideal patriotism "must be based not upon a consciousness of homogeneity but upon a respect for variation."[8] For Addams, difference was the basis for a new kind of cosmopolitan American identity, and physical education offered a tool for maintaining its moral standards amid the threat of an emergent youth culture. Gilman, in contrast, was taken aback by what she described to a friend as "all the stress of this mixed living" at Hull-House.[9] In 1898 she disparagingly referred to those who utilized the settlement's resources as "a vortex of nations" that, as her biographer Cynthia J. Davis put it, Gilman would have preferred to "avoid being sucked up into."[10] Gilman saw physical education as a biopolitical tool that women could wield to standardize "deviant" bodies in order to create a more homogenous nation. Reading Gilman's and Addams's approaches in tandem thus reveals a central tension for turn-of-the-century physical education. As professionally trained experts took on responsibility for diverse populations, they had to determine whether physical activity should be a means of expressing differences or eradicating them.

For both Addams and Gilman, the authority many women assumed as professional physical educators was an extension of what Caroll Smith-Rosenberg calls the role of "public mothers," who, through their reform efforts, "cared for hundreds, even thousands" of children.[11] Indeed, the maternal responsibility of caregiving was central to both Addams's and Gilman's politics.[12] In her 1911 lecture "Woman and the State," later republished as "If Men Were Seeking the Franchise," Addams briefly constructs a utopian vision of a country with an inverted status quo. She imagines "wise women governing the State with the same care they had always put into the management of their families," deliberating on whether or not to enfranchise their male counterparts who "do not really know how tender and delicate children are, and might put them to work in factories."[13] Gilman would later expand on this thought experiment in her *Herland* (1915). The novel, which depicts an all-female, expertly governed nation's encounter with male interlopers, who are stunned by both the national standard of health and the advanced child-rearing methods that ensure it. In the spirit of the Progressive Era in which they lived and wrote, both Addams's and Gilman's imagined societies represented a higher standard of health. These nations run by women could beget healthier children, and the professionalization of physical education played an important role in women's gaining such authority over children's health. "Every public school teacher," Gilman wrote in 1912, "is a government official, she has been in politics for some time."[14] Indeed, as women like as Bancroft assumed responsibility for the physical education not only of their own classes of students but of entire districts, the field emerged as a powerful tool for managing the health of the population.

Addams's and Gilman's theories of physical education represent an important dimension of women's health politics at the turn of the century, a period that has often been defined by the eugenic feminism of prominent activists such as Margaret Sanger and Victoria Woodhull, who championed selective reproduction as a strategy for racial evolution. Gilman, too, was associated with the eugenics movement, and scholars have primarily addressed her efforts to position white women as agents of racial nationalism by emphasizing her ideas about reproduction.[15] This is only part of the story: Gilman also insisted on the importance of "improvement" after birth. "Unless the first years are rightly treated," she insisted, "we lose in wrong education much of the fruit of right breeding."[16] Addams, too, was invested in human plasticity and saw it as women's responsibility to create optimal conditions for human development. "During those first years on Halsted Street," she writes of Hull-House's opening, "nothing was more painfully clear than the fact that pliable human nature is relentlessly pressed upon by its physical environment."[17] Addams and the experts she hired worked to carefully control young people's environments, helping them become what she once called a "better type."[18] Far from redressing readings of Gilman's and her contemporaries' eugenic commitments, turning to physical education brings into focus a broader set of practices through which US-born white women varyingly expressed and negotiated eugenic impulses. The rise of white women's public "mother-work" at the turn of the century was driven by racial anxieties, and assimilation was often central to their caregiving efforts.[19] By applying their maternal authority to the existing bodies of children and adolescents, these women showed that the population could be shaped, as Gilman put it, by "more than mothers."[20]

Immigration and "Biological Engineering" at the Turn of the Century

Over the course of the decades during which Addams and Gilman developed their distinct approaches to physical education, the composition of the US body politic changed dramatically. Between 1880 and 1920, the country's foreign-born population doubled, reaching nearly 14 million people.[21] The majority of these new arrivals hailed from Southern and Eastern Europe.[22] This period of mass immigration coincided with the rise of eugenics, a field that put the bodies and characters of the foreign-born and their children under intense scrutiny by physicians and social reformers alike. For immigration officials at Ellis Island especially, intersecting ideas about race and disability positioned many potential arrivals as "defective" threats to the national genetic pool.[23] Assessments of physical health were a crucial tool in determining who was and was not allowed to enter the country. Jay Dolmage has demonstrated that movement through Ellis Island was highly choreographed, ensuring that immigration agents had ample opportunity to assess the arrivals' bodies. Victor Safford, an Ellis Island medical officer, described his task as "to detect poorly built, defective or broken down human beings."[24] He did this not only in the formal context of an examination but also by observing how arrivals moved through the facility. He recalled, "we used to like to have passengers . . . make two right angle turns," which "helped to bring out imperfections in muscular coordination."[25] By 1904, muscular quality was a matter of policy, and "poor physique" became an official category of exclusion.

Outside the confines of Ellis Island, eugenicists feared that medical assessments alone could not adequately protect the United States from the threat certain racial groups posed to the population's health. Robert DeCourcey Ward, who cofounded the Immigration Restriction League in 1894, later declared, "There can be absolutely no doubt that the recent change in the races of our immigrants will profoundly affect the character of the future American race" and produce negative "physical and mental changes."[26] In his widely read volume *Heredity in Relation to Eugenics* (1911), Charles Davenport similarly warned that without increased restrictions, "the United States will, on account of the great influx of blood from South-Eastern Europe, rapidly become darker in pigmentation, smaller in stature, more mercurial, more attached to music and art, more given to crimes of larceny, kidnapping, assault, murder, rape, and sex-immorality."[27] Both Ward and Davenport were convinced that protecting the physiological makeup of Americans could not be accomplished by screening for individual "defects," but instead required population-level exclusions.

As Davenport's declaration makes clear, the threat of "poor physique" was urgent for eugenicists because it reflected a host of negative qualities that were deemed transmissible. In 1905, Bureau of Immigration commissioner general F. P. Sargent explained that an immigrant with a "poor physique" was "not likely to become a desirable citizen, but also very likely to transmit his undesirable qualities to his offspring," who "will reproduce, often in an exaggerated degree, the physical degeneracy of their parents."[28] As Douglas Baynton has shown, criminality was chief among these "undesirable qualities." As early as 1898, prominent professor of medicine Eugene Talbot claimed that "crime is hereditary, a tendency which is, in most cases, associated with bodily defect."[29] Ward similarly insisted that by failing to adequately restrict immigration, the United States was essentially "legalizing the begetting of criminal children."[30] Leading eugenicists argued that physical, mental, and moral health were determined primarily by biological rather than environmental factors. As Immigration Restriction League cofounder Prescot F. Hall put it, "you cannot make bad stock into good stock by changing its meridian" or geographic location "any more than you can . . . make a mongrel into a fine dog by teaching it tricks."[31] Though suggesting that recent immigrants and their descendants may learn to perform American identity, Hall derided these as mere "tricks." The composition of the body itself, he implied, is the only true mark of an ideal American.

While eugenicists insisted on the heritability of immigrants' physical "defects" and associated character traits, an alternative theory was emerging from an immigrant himself: the renowned anthropologist Franz Boas, a German Jew who arrived in the United States in 1887. According to Boas, environmental factors were key in producing perceived social differences between racial groups. In 1894, he claimed that "historical events appear to have been much more potent in leading races to civilization than their faculty."[32] Roughly a decade later, he examined whether physical differences might be similarly contingent. From 1908 to 1910, the US Immigration Commission funded Boas's research on the physiological impact of immigration. After measuring the heads of approximately 18,000 immigrants and their children living in urban settings, even Boas himself was surprised to discover differences between children and their parents.[33] In particular, he determined that head shape—previously considered a fixed trait that differentiated European groups—was not simply hereditary, but was environmentally contingent. When the US Immigration Commission presented Boas's research to Congress in December 1909, they raised the possibility that, if head shape was now proven mutable, "may it not be that other characteristics may be as easily modified and that there may be a rapid assimilation of widely varying nationalities and races to something that may well be called an American type?"[34] Within a matter of weeks, the story of what many headlines called "An American Type" appeared in publications across the country.[35] The study had immense consequences for physiological understandings of race and assimilation.[36] As Boas wrote in his official report, "all evidence is now in favor of a great plasticity of human types."[37] Like eugenicists, Boas saw the body as a proxy for a host of traits—"types" were not exclusively physical. "We are compelled to conclude," he wrote, "that when these features of the body change, the whole bodily and mental make-up of the immigrants may change."[38]

By this logic, the immigrant was not a threat to American physiological standards but might instead be shaped to meet them.

The notion that immigrants' bodies were plastic quickly drew attention from physical educators. At the turn of the century, physical education was establishing itself as a rigorous human science in its own right, and it did so in part by adopting a stance on biological difference that bridged eugenic determinism and that of "euthenists" like Boas who saw the immigrant's capacity for improvement under changed circumstances. Like eugenicists, educators envisioned a standardized American physique, though they followed Boas in expanding who they believed was capable of embodying it.[39] An important distinguishing feature of physical education, though, was that experts not only recognized the human capacity for improvement—they also claimed they knew how to facilitate such transformation. As Martha Verbrugge has shown, physical educators saw classifications such as sex, race, and age as a matter of physiology, and they believed that "'education through the physical' cultivated the values and traits that a democratic, industrial society required."[40] As an applied science, then, physical education sought to improve the American body and, by extension, its moral character.

Leading this charge was Dr. Charles Ward Crampton, the director of physical training of the public schools of New York City (where he was Jessie Hubbel Bancroft's longtime supervisor), whom Boas credits with "ably assist[ing]" his research among immigrant children in the city.[41] Crampton clearly embraced Boas's claims about human malleability. In his 1922 volume *The Pedagogy of Physical Training*, Crampton reflects on the evolution of the field over the two preceding decades. He describes a "growing unanimity of ideals in physical education."[42] "America," he writes, "is making its own system" of physical training—perhaps one intended to produce the much-celebrated possibility of an "American type." Wary of the United States' "increasing constitutional inferiority," Crampton calls for physical education as a means of "adapting" the nation to the effects of modern life.[43] "This is biological engineering," he declares, "a new profession, in the ranks of which physical training teachers take their place."[44] Because the field is concerned "with the health and vigor of the human race," Crampton continues, "it has assumed a responsibility in the maintenance of the very structure of civilization."[45] Crampton thus explicitly establishes physical education as a biopolitical endeavor and a tool for enacting corporeal transformation at the level of the population.

Crampton's colleague and the nation's most famous physical educator, Dr. Dudley Allen Sargent, who directed both Harvard's Hemenway Gymnasium and the Boston Normal School of Physical Training (later renamed the Sargent School of Physical Training), more explicitly incorporated eugenic insights into his theories. Sargent, whose library included volumes by Charles Darwin as well as Darwin's cousin, Francis Galton, who coined the term "eugenics," shared the anxieties of those working to restrict immigration.[46] In *Physical Education* (1906), he asserts that "the immigrants who began to come to America about the middle of the last century represented a much poorer quality of stock physically than those who had preceded them."[47] These new arrivals, he argues, have "undoubtedly impaired the physical status of our people as a whole" by lowering the quality of "the average physique."[48] Like many of his contemporaries, Sargent believed that physical deterioration would produce a corresponding decline in American morality. He insisted on "the importance of a good physique as a basis for a high moral and intellectual life" and claimed that "criminals, dullards, and the mentally defective" possessed "very poor physiques."[49]

Unlike many eugenicists, though, Sargent was adamant that desirable traits could be cultivated through physical education. In 1900, he insisted on "the value of physical training as an essential prerequisite to the attainment of the highest intellectual results in a school, a college, a community, or a race."[50] For Sargent, the training of physical educators was essential to achieving this elevated standard. As he wrote in his autobiography, "my great work . . . would be for nothing, unless I could supply people who were trained to teach the new method."[51] He argued that "the nations that have given the most attention to the care of the body," a group he hoped the United States might join, "have not only been of a superior quality physically but also have invariably attained the greatest mental preeminence."[52] For Sargent and the legions of physical educators he trained and inspired, eugenic differentiations among races held true, but the environment, too, was predictive of character.

Though establishing itself as a specialized science, physical educators' theories were not relegated to professional networks alone. Gilman, for instance, read about Sargent's pedagogy in his mentor William Blaikie's popular volume *How to Get Strong and How to Stay So* (1878), a book she cherished. As a young woman, she also joined a gymnasium that she described as "thoroughly stocked with apparatus selected by Dr. Sargent of Harvard University."[53] Throughout her career, she continued to write about Sargent, whom she called "the wise and successful promoter of physical education in this country."[54] Addams, too, encountered Sargent in her efforts to cultivate the bodies of immigrant children. Rose Gyles, who directed the

Hull-House gymnasium for decades beginning with its 1893 opening and whose work Addams greatly revered, was a graduate of Sargent's Hemenway Gymnasium. In 1916, when Addams was president of the Woman's Peace Party (of which Gilman was also a member), the party sent a woman to study under Sargent in order to prepare materials for a "compulsory physical training bill" they hoped Congress might pass.[55] Both Addams's and Gilman's visions of national physical education were shaped by the field's core tension between eugenic determinism and a belief that the ideal American physique could be cultivated. Reflecting the "improvement" ethos of the Progressive Era during which they lived, both reformers reckoned with difference while striving toward an optimized future. Despite this shared position and their overlapping careers, the two came to wholly different conclusions about how best to attend to the immigrant child's body and find a place for it in the American body politic.

Cosmopolitanism and Expertise at Hull-House

In 1889, Addams and Ellen Gates Starr established the Hull-House settlement in Chicago, where recent immigration from Southern and Eastern Europe over the previous decade had expanded the population by more than 600,000, making it the nation's second largest city.[56] During Hull-House's early years, 78 percent of Chicago residents were either foreign-born or first-generation Americans, and the settlement "residents" from middle- and upper-class backgrounds lived alongside these families, holding classes, forming clubs, and providing neighborly support.[57] Hull-House was run primarily by women, and much of the settlement's activity focused on the well-being of children.[58] Whether in the nursery, in the gymnasium, or on the playground, specially trained Hull-House residents attended to children's health at all stages of development.

One of the settlement's first endeavors was a nursery, which began informally when working mothers started leaving their children with Addams and the other residents. Though she herself performed it, Addams later derided this supervision as "so-called care," and she quickly recruited more "systematic supervision."[59] In her 1892 essay "The Objective Value of a Social Settlement," Addams makes clear that the children are now in expert hands. She describes "a young lady who has had kindergarten training" as responsible for a formal crèche.[60] The kindergarten class, too, she reports, is led by "a professional teacher."[61] Both quickly grew in size and were moved to a nearby cottage later that year. In 1895, the settlement erected a designated "Children's

Building" to house both programs and, in 1908, moved them to the Mary Crane Nursery.[62]

These early childcare programs mirrored the structure of the settlement's gymnastics classes, which were designed for older children and young adults. Hull-House opened its gymnasium in 1893 with Rose Gyles as director. A graduate of Sargent's Harvard program, Gyles was a certified expert, and Addams took great pride in the quality of the gymnastics program. In a 1904 letter, she commended Gyles for her rigorous approach, writing that "there is certainly no department [at Hull-House] which goes on more smoothly or with higher standards."[63] Outside the gymnasium, Gyles brought her expertise to the playground, which was also erected in 1893. Establishing the importance of her supervision, Gyles told the *Chicago Daily Tribune* in 1894 that because the children who visited the Hull-House playground "do not know how to play," "we try to keep someone with the children during the day as much as possible to teach them games."[64] Play was a serious educational endeavor at Hull-House. Throughout the 1910s, Neva Boyd, who founded the Chicago School for Playground Workers in 1911, supervised student fieldwork at the Hull-House playground and taught "playground courses" on pedagogy and play in the settlement's gymnasium.[65] By 1920, Boyd had fully relocated her work to Hull-House, where she established the Recreation Training School.

When describing these educational venues, Addams foregrounded the expert knowledge of Hull-House residents, but she also emphasized her pupils' distinct needs and perspectives. Like John Dewey, her friend and repeated Hull-House visitor, Addams championed a model of "progressive education" that reflected the porous boundary between learning environments and civil society.[66] For Addams, this framework translated to physical education as well. Addams saw children not only as beneficiaries of physical education, but also as collaborators. In a 1908 address before the National Education Association, Addams held up the educational theorist (and early physical education advocate) Johann Heinrich Pestalozzi as a pedagogical ideal. She describes his work managing an orphanage in Switzerland, where, rather than assume the children's needs, Pestalozzi "was obliged to appeal to the children for help; to follow their lead," and, as a result, "he was put into the very best possible attitude for making educational discoveries."[67] This willingness to learn from the children in his care offered Addams a model for educators. "Perhaps in time," she suggests, "educators who are assisted by the devoted parents may come to recognize ['mentally deficient'] children as possible contributors toward the solution of the public-school problems."[68] Though here she writes about disabled children rather than immigrants, her claim that in order to address "the problem," one must "consider it from the point of view of the child" reflects a remarkably anti-eugenic stance on the role of education in caring for those deemed outside the norm.[69]

If effective pedagogy involved "keep[ing] in mind the child's suggestions for his own needs," Hull-House focused on how these needs were shaped by pupils' diverse cultural backgrounds.[70] "Exercise and play," Shannon Jackson notes, sometimes served as "a physical means of assimilation" at Hull-House, but they could also be "an expression of cultural identification."[71] In *Democracy and Social Ethics* (1902), Addams describes children of immigrants who, until they reach school age, learn from relatives using methods that reflect their heritage. Of the child's ancestors, she speculates, "open air and activity of body have been the inevitable accompaniments of all their experiences. Yet the first thing that the boy must do when he reaches school is to sit still, at least part of the time."[72] Romanticizing her immigrant neighbors' family origins, Addams presents these European approaches as more embodied and healthful than sedentary American norms. Addams thus frames her investment in expanded physical education instruction not as an imposition of American standards, but as an effort to meet what she sees as children's culturally inherited needs.

Addams's resistance to overly standardized pedagogy mirrored her concerns about overgeneralizations regarding immigrants. In a 1919 essay on "Americanization," Addams declares that "the application of a collective judgment in regard to aliens in the United States is particularly stupid."[73] "The twenty-seven million people of foreign birth living among us," she continues, "are in fact more highly differentiated from each other by race, tradition, religion, and European background than the rest of us."[74] In her memoir *Twenty Years at Hull-House* (1910), Addams reveals that the heterogeneity among immigrants was a lesson she learned at least in part from children. She recalls, "That first kindergarten was a constant source of education to us. We were much surprised to find social distinctions even among its lambs."[75] By celebrating—and, at times, idealizing—the diverse needs of her diverse pupils, Addams pursued what Tova Cooper describes as "a progressive vision of citizenship education that validates cultural difference rather than seeking its erasure."[76] Addams saw the gymnasium, for example, as an opportunity for Greek cultural expression. In *Twenty Years*, she writes that "The Greek immigrants form large classes and are eager to reproduce the remnants of old methods of wrestling, and other bits of classic lore which they still possess."[77] Addams's student-centered pedagogy reflected the settlement's broader ethos. If "Hull-House was soberly opened on the theory that the dependence of classes on each other is reciprocal," then the settlement's educational programs, too, were structured by Addams's belief in a reciprocal dynamic between teachers and students.[78]

Addams also saw physical education as an opportunity for cross-cultural exchange, and she articulates her cosmopolitan theory of play explicitly in "Recreation as a Public Function in Urban Communities" (1912). In this essay published in the *American Journal of Sociology*, Addams asserts that recreational spaces including playgrounds, gymnasiums, and swimming pools provide an ideal environment in which to forge a new kind of American identity. "There is no doubt," she argues, "that the future patriotism of America must depend not so much upon conformity as upon respect for variety, and nowhere can this be inculcated as it can in the public recreation centers."[79] Addams explains the unique relationship between recreation and heterogeneity:

> As immigrants to America work together in factories, every effort is made that they should conform to a common standard; as they walk upon the street they make painful exertion to approach a prevailing mode in dress; only on the playground or in the recreation center do they find that variety is prized, that distinctive folklore and national customs as well as individual initiative are at a premium. They meet together and enjoy each other's national dances and games, and as the sense of comradeship and pleasure grows, they are able to express, as nowhere else, that sense of being unlike one's fellows which is at the basis of all progress.[80]

Physical activity here is not the stifling, assimilationist tool implemented at the Carlisle Indian Industrial School, but rather a cultural antidote to the uniformity that immigrants perform in other public spaces. The opportunity to partake in one another's traditional dances and games, Addams insists, will heighten immigrants' awareness of what differentiates them. Rather than alienate them from one another, though, this process will forge "comradeship," "progress," and ultimately "a higher type of citizenship."[81]

When Addams writes that this "higher type" of citizenship is being "nursed" in recreation centers, she signals her commitment to supervised activity. Even as she argues that immigrants will teach each other traditional games and dances, she still insists on the importance of American expertise. Because, as she puts it, the "pain and confusion" that accompanies culture clashes in diverse populations "sometimes intensifies . . . into a pathological condition," it is "necessary to put it under the direction of skilled instructors and to provide places where it may be carried on normally."[82] Addams's ideal form of physical education offers a kind of regulated cosmopolitanism. Though she does not position educators as the sole sources of knowledge on the playground or in the gymnasium, she does imbue them with unique disciplinary power. She suggests that potentially "pathological" unmediated or improperly supervised recreation does pose a eugenically coded threat: delinquency.

Though she embraced cosmopolitanism, Addams was not immune to the logic of "improvement" that pervaded Progressive-Era reform movements as well as physical education discourse. She makes this tension between her reverence for difference and this definition of progress plain in a chapter of *Twenty Years* entitled "Immigrants and Their Children." "One thing seemed clear in regard to entertaining immigrants," Addams writes, "to preserve and keep whatever of value their past life contained and to bring them in contact with a better type of Americans."[83] Addams locates value in immigrant knowledge and experience as well as in US-born women's ability to determine that value, but she ultimately hopes that the experts she has enlisted might help mold the children of immigrants into not only what the Immigration Commission called an "American type" but also a "better type."[84] As the anxieties about "pathological" behavior expressed in "Recreation as a Public Function" make clear, Addams did see physical education as an opportunity to intervene in immigrants' moral development. She was convinced that "the number of arrests among juvenile delinquents falls off surprisingly in a neighborhood where . . . a park has been established."[85] "Give the children a chance to play," Addams insisted, "and they will not become criminals."[86] In addition to her cosmopolitan "respect for variety," then, Addams embraced physical education's promise of promoting moral improvement through bodily management in the face of rising concerns about juvenile delinquency and vice among the urban poor.

Unlike the eugenicists, Addams did not see morality as racially determined. On the contrary, she argued that it was the conditions of living in American cities that drove young immigrants to alcohol, crime, and sex—all of which were considered interrelated threats to American moral standards. "The overt disobedience to the law on the part of a child brought into the Juvenile Court," she argued, "is regarded as a symptom not only that something is wrong with the child himself, but also that something is wrong with his home, his school and neighborhood surroundings."[87] According to Addams, "the conditions surrounding these young people" and not their biological makeup was the source of their deviance.[88]

Addams did, however, share eugenicists' belief that physical health and moral character were intimately connected. In a 1913 entry in *Ladies' Home Journal*, Addams details the ways in which the United States renders immigrants "crippled and depleted."[89] She describes a number of labor-related injuries and also adds that immigrants are subject to "a higher rate of death" and "increasing insanity" than other Americans due to unsafe working conditions, contaminated food and drink, and the "the nervous strain of maladjustment" to this new locale.[90] For Addams, the solution to immigrant inferiority is not removal or exclusion as it was for immigration officials, but public health measures. She proposes "a National public health service" that would provide "inspection and supervision of those labor camps and crowded lodging houses in which thousands of immigrants who come to us in good health and with decent habits so often contract disease and vicious practices."[91] Addams proposes that government intervention will provide improved morality along with physical health. She urges readers that, "Unless some systematic effort is made on their behalf these large groups of future citizens will not only lose their own health and virtue, but also will become a menace to the entire community."[92] She positions her advocacy as not just a benevolent effort on behalf of the immigrant, but as an attempt to protect other, presumably virtuous citizens from the threat of immoral interlopers.

In addition to her "National public health service" of inspectors, Addams imagined physical education as a means of promoting immigrant health and, as a result, morality. Without organized play, Addams argued, Americans "are spoiling and maiming" children "by giving them no proper chance of development."[93] She argued that young people desperately needed alternatives to the dance halls, amusement parks, and theaters that "present[ed] endless opportunities for enticing young people into wrongdoing."[94] This she saw as the responsibility of educators, whom she chastised "for neglecting to give children instruction in play when one sees the unregulated amusement parks which are apparently so dangerous."[95] As she put it in her 1909 book *The Spirit of Youth and the City Streets*, "recreation alone can stifle the lust for vice."[96] Addams argues that because the government has failed to "organize play," the youthful "love of pleasure" that play might satiate has devolved into "all sorts of malignant and vicious appetites."[97] For example, she cites "an eminent alienist of Chicago" who claims that overexposure to the theater has produced "mental disorder" in "neurotic children."[98] As an alternative, Addams proposes "public games easily carried out in a park or athletic field," which might satisfy the desire for "imaginative material constantly supplied by the theater" and also promote health through "the activity which the cramped muscles of the town dweller so sorely need."[99] According to Addams, supervised athletic play could provide physically healthful exercise while simultaneously regulating the imagination so degraded by the theater.

Indeed, Addams saw the Hull-House recreation facilities as alternatives to immoral leisure activities. In *Twenty Years*, she reports that "Our gymnasium has been filled with large and enthusiastic classes for eighteen years in spite of the popularity of dancing and other possible substitutes."[100] Athletics didn't simply keep young people out of dance halls—they also insisted that participants be morally upright. "The Settlement," Addams explains, "strives for that type of gymnastics which is at least partly a matter of character, for that training which presupposes abstinence and the curbing of impulse."[101] James Salazar has demonstrated that, as an extension of her cosmopolitan sensibilities, Addams sought to cultivate "transnational character" by creating "intercultural spaces" within the settlement house, including the gymnasium.[102] At the same time, though, Addams signaled the disciplining nature of athletics by demanding the "management of impulse" and promoting "athletic contests in which the mind of the contestant must be vigilant to keep the body closely to the rules of the game."[103] Adhering to these rules, Addams implied, was not so different from abiding by the law. Indeed, in lieu of unregulated commercial amusements run for profit, Addams proposed "model dance halls under municipal control" as well as "more parks, properly policed."[104] In fact, during the first decade at Hull-House, activity on the playground was not only overseen by Gyles, Boyd, and other women teachers; it was also managed by a police officer, whose presence makes clear the extent to which the insistence on supervised, structured play was bound up with other disciplinary mechanisms.[105]

Though Addams's efforts to regulate recreation seemingly contradict her reverence for culturally specific forms of expression, the two aspects of her thinking are complementary. Addams celebrated young people's efforts to embrace their parents' cultures of origin, and worried that the emergent youth culture would displace not only American moral norms but also the traditions and values of immigrant parents. In her address "The Public School and the Immigrant Child," Addams cites research showing that "while the number of arrests of immigrants is smaller than the arrests of native born Americans, the number of arrests among children of immigrants is twice as large as the number of arrests among the children of native born Americans."[106] These data suggest that criminality is not an essential trait, but an environmental product. Like Boas, Addams was interested especially in the differences between immigrants and their offspring, though rather than echo the news media's celebration of these children's Americanization, Addams feared that becoming estranged from their foreign-born parents would leave them "without a sufficient rudder and power of self-direction, into the perilous business of living."[107] According to Addams, maintaining a connection to their parents' culture was crucial to preventing delinquency in immigrant children, and physical education could give them an opportunity to practice embodying Old World values.

As such, Addams promoted cosmopolitanism as a means of increasing physical education's impact. In a 1908 essay in the philanthropy publication *Charities and the Commons*, she recalls "a long summer day in one of our large playing fields" in Chicago filled not only with "kindergarten games" and "athletic sports" but also with "Italians, Lithuanians, Norwegians, and a dozen other nationalities reproducing their old dances and festivals."[108] According to Addams, "These old forms of dancing which have been worked out in many lands and through long experience, safeguard unwary and dangerous expressions and yet afford a vehicle through which the joy of youth may flow."[109] By virtue of being "old," she suggests, traditional dances offer an antidote to the unrestrained youth culture that she sees as tainting the morals of immigrant children.

Remarkably, Addams invokes eugenics when she describes the "forms" of the "old dances" as "those which lie at the basis of all good breeding, forms which at once express and restrain, urge forward and set limits."[110] Just as the Hull-House gymnastics training prioritized "abstinence and the curbing of impulse," so too do traditional dances regulate potentially unwieldy desire in order to create a subject who is likely to "breed" responsibly.[111] Indeed, though she did not figure specific racial groups as "unfit" for reproduction, Addams did advocate for sexual restraint as a eugenic measure. She saw the "children's rights" movement as "allied" with "the new science of eugenics" insofar as she believed in "a child's right to be well born and to start in life with its tiny body free from disease."[112] In particular, Addams was concerned about sexually transmitted diseases, which she saw as "responsible for race deterioration" since "the survivors among these afflicted children infect their contemporaries and hand on the evil heritage to another generation."[113] The possibility of unrestrained sex that the dance halls and similar arenas posed thus made unsupervised recreation a distinctly eugenic threat.[114] For Addams, then, wholesome physical activity was not only an opportunity for intercultural exchange; it was also an anchor to the Old World traditions she hoped would distract from more indecent activities. Supervised play, Addams ultimately argued, promoted diversity while also diverting deviance.

Gilman, Eugenics, and "Child Culture"

While Addams saw physical education as a means of instilling healthful and moral behaviors in diverse young people, her contemporary and friend Charlotte Perkins Gilman took a more biological approach to human "improvement." After the two met in 1894 at the California Woman's Congress, which Gilman helped organize, Addams described Gilman as "the one bright spot in San Francisco" and invited her to spend part of the following year as a resident at Hull-House.[115] Gilman resided at Hull-House from approximately September until early December of 1895—the same year that Hull-House erected its Children's Building.[116] Over the next few years, Gilman worked the lecture circuit, but she often returned to Chicago. From 1897 to 1899, she frequented lectures, club meetings, and meals at what she once called "the greatest 'Social Settlement' in America" as she continued to develop her theories.[117] In her autobiography, *The Living of Charlotte Perkins Gilman*, she recalled that during her Chicago years, "the social philosophy I was teaching included . . . [the] specialization of women as essential to the improvement of marriage, motherhood, domestic industry, and racial improvement; with much on advance in child culture."[118]

Gilman shared Crampton's view of physical education as a method of "biological engineering," and she hoped women might take on this responsibility for racial progress. As Michelle Ann Abate and Salazar each have argued, Gilman insisted that exercise would transform women's bodies along with their social roles by enabling them to produce more desirable offspring.[119] Such expertise in exercise also enabled women who did *not* reproduce to play a role in forming a homogeneous, superior nation. Though she shared eugenicists' goals, Gilman was skeptical of their methods, which she dismissed as a form of "man's talk" that overemphasized breeding and overlooked other processes (such as education) that determined health.[120] In a 1910 essay on "Prize Children," she mocks "those who come to us talking largely of eugenics; wanting us to breed super-men and super-women," explaining that "this method of breeding and selection . . . has to be accompanied by a ruthless slaughter of the unfit, and takes thousands upon thousands of years."[121] Though it is unclear whether her skepticism is rooted in the violence or the impracticality of eugenics, Gilman proposes instead to "improve the species after it is born."[122] When she describes women's "racial importance as makers of men," Gilman refers not only to reproductive labor, but also to the work of child-rearing.[123] This approach was grounded in a Lamarckian theory of heredity that figured acquired traits as transmissible.[124] For Gilman, "the life process we call education" was best understood as "the replenishment and development of the race."[125] Physical education, she suggested, was as predictive of both national and individual physical "fitness" as parental biology, and was thus similarly in need of intervention. Indeed, across both her fictional and sociological writings, Gilman equips US-born, white women experts with immense biopolitical influence by imagining their capacity to shape future generations.

Like Addams, Gilman readily embraced the professionalization of physical education. As a teenager, she attended a lecture by Dr. Mary J. Studley that she later recalled left "an indelible impression," prompting her to pursue "every kind of attainable physical exercise."[126] Studley's health manual, *What Our Girls Ought to Know* (1878), may also have shaped Gilman's investment in expert child-rearing. "Do not, I pray you," Studley implores future teachers, "offer yourself as a guide for other people's children without this preparation. If you do, you put yourself in the ranks of those who hang out a doctor's sign without ever having made a study of the profession of medicine."[127] Another of Gilman's major influences, Sargent's mentor William Blaikie, wrote in *How to Get Strong and How to Stay So* (1879) that "men like Sargent, strict disciplinarians, trained physicians, and practical gymnasts as well are far too scarce among us. . . . Let the school commissioners . . . insist that each teacher shall forthwith obtain the knowledge requisite to properly instruct and bring forward every pupil in his or her class."[128] As she came of age in the late nineteenth century, then, Gilman was exposed to physical education as a distinctly professional science, and she continued to return to the discipline for inspiration throughout her career.

Such professional expertise was crucial to Gilman's critique of "the divine instinct of maternity."[129] Gilman was highly skeptical of the widespread perception of motherhood as an identity rooted in sentimentality rather than an occupation requiring the studious acquisition of scientific knowledge.[130] In her sociological text, *Women and Economics* (1898), she includes motherhood among the many devalued forms of women's labor and advocates for a more scientifically informed approach to child-rearing. "The education of young women," she remarks, "has no department of maternity . . . this most important and wonderful of human functions is left from age to age in the hands of absolutely untaught women" with "neither education for that wonderful work nor experience."[131] Like her aunt, Catharine Beecher, whose ideas appear in chapter 2, Gilman insists on the importance of recognizing women's domestic labor as a specialized occupation.[132] She points out that "before a man enters a trade, art, or profession, he studies it . . . qualifies himself for the duties he is to undertake," and she proposes that women be held to a similar standard of preparation for their work.[133] Gilman argued that "pedagogy" could and should be "taught as a science."[134] In her 1909 story, "A Garden of Babies," published in the magazine *Success* in 1909, the narrator describes her sister, Jessie, who took a course in "baby nursing" before opening a childcare facility reminiscent of the Hull-House crèche.[135] Jessie takes on only "trained assistants," who she requires to "learn a lot of elementary physiology, hygiene, sanitation."[136] She condemns women who rely on "instinct," a fiction she claims "is accountable for thousands of little graves—thousands of blind, crippled, sick, imbecile, degenerate children."[137] As the language of disability here reveals, uninformed child-rearing poses a eugenic threat that Gilman believed proper training could combat.

Gilman depicts the process of becoming a specialist in children's development in her 1910 novel *The Crux* when the protagonist, Vivian Lane, begins an apprenticeship under "a stalwart instructress, a large-boned, calm-eyed Swedish woman," who "is perfectly reliable and an excellent teacher."[138] Vivian is cautioned early on in her training that "you'll have to go through [the children's] little exercises with them," making it clear that Vivian, too, has much to learn from this expert.[139] Vivian, who early in the novel is described as "read[ing] the queerest things—doctor's books and works on pedagoggy [sic]," appears uniquely suited for such training.[140] Her apprenticeship proves successful; after a "season in Mrs. Johnson's gymnastic class," Vivian has learned to approach her work "patiently and steadily," and she receives a promotion in the form of a salary, entering the ranks of professional physical educators.[141] Rather than simply develop her own body in order to become a eugenically fit mother, Vivian trains physically and mentally for her maternally coded profession.

Gilman did not reject the notion of maternal "instinct" entirely, however, but argued instead that was an exceedingly rare trait possessed by "only about one in twenty."[142] In Gilman's writing, expertise itself emerges as a eugenic ideal. Though these uniquely suited individuals still require "full training, long experience and a proper environment," they do possess a "special gift a high order of intellect, and a real talent" for the work.[143] In *Concerning Children* (1903), Gilman goes further to insist that "babies and small children ought to have the society of the very best people instead of the society of such low-grade women as we can hire to be nurses in our homes."[144] She laments that "we confide [white children] to the care of distinctly lower races, as in the South with its negro nurses," but "we do not yet consider . . . whether a servant is a good educator."[145] Here, the explicitly racist dimensions of Gilman's white feminist worldview converge with her concerns about expertise. Echoing the antebellum derision of racialized women who worked as "domestics" that I described in chapters 2 and 3 (including the attitudes of her aunt, Catharine), she asserts a narrow class of white women represented by characters like Jessie and Vivian as "the best people" to transform the body politic.

Gilman illustrates the interaction between inherent fitness for child-rearing and thorough professional training in *Moving the Mountain*, a novel she released serially in her self-published magazine *The Forerunner* in 1911. Set in the 1940s, *Moving the Mountain* imagines a future in which the country has implemented a "department of maternity." Training in motherhood is not a curricular requirement for all female students but rather one of many "specialties" available. In Gilman's utopian vision, "those women best fitted for the work" of child-rearing "had given eager, devoted lives to it and built up a new science of Humaniculture."[146] In the hyperregulated eugenic future Gilman imagines, "a clean bill of health" is required by applicants for marriage licenses and "any woman can be a mother—if she's normal," but being a "child-culturist" requires a diploma.[147] When one character explains to an outsider that "no woman was allowed to care for her children without proof of capacity" and credentialing by "the Department of Child Culture—the Government," the term "capacity" refers to an ability that is equally innate and cultivated.[148]

Gilman presents the effects of expert child-rearing as a complement to selective reproduction. In this society where "health—physical purity—was made a practical ideal," the youth, as one character puts it, are both "clean-born, vigorous children, inheriting strength and purity" and benefiting from "special conditions for child-culture."[149] By "conditions," she means not only methods, but also facilities, as "we build for babies now."[150] Much of the child culture outlined in *Moving the Mountain* centers on specially designed environments. All children are reared in "child gardens," elaborated versions of the facility depicted in "A Garden of Babies" that invoke the Hull-House Children's Building and, later, the Mary Crane Nursery. In Gilman's novel, these spaces are engineered to support and maximize children's physical exploration: the toddlers "rolled and tumbled on smooth mattresses; pulled themselves up and swung back and forth on large, soft horizontal ropes fastened within reach."[151] The experts in "Humaniculture" clearly possess the scientific expertise Gilman valued in physical educators—they've tailored children's environments to their developmental stages: "As they grew larger and more competent, their playgrounds were more extensive and varied."[152] The opportunities these facilities present for physical education underpin the foundation of their pedagogy. "The main joy" for students "was in the use of their own little bodies," and the "atmosphere" of the educational environment was defined by "growth, exercise, and joy."[153]

Gilman elaborates on such corporeal pedagogy in her 1915 novel *Herland*, in which the citizens of the titular all-female nation are descended parthenogenetically from a single ancestral mother.[154] Rosemarie Garland-Thomson argues that *Herland* depicts a standardized citizenry achieved largely through positive eugenics; assessments of each woman determine the number of children she will bear, and some are discouraged from reproduction altogether.[155] Their idealized physiques, however, are also produced through education, which the Herlanders call "our highest art."[156] The novel's male narrator, Van, refers to the "athletic, light, and powerful" Herlanders as "experts," with "trained athletic bodies," suggesting a broader system of cultivation.[157] Indeed, he reports that they've developed "a most excellent system" of physical culture.[158] The Herlanders are not simply "born better," but also made so—the women "train out" as well as "breed out, when possible, the lowest types."[159]

This training is all-encompassing and begins in early childhood. In a civic society that Lorraine Krall McCrary explains represents "family practiced on a large scale," the enrollment of young children in state-run care facilities does not displace familial love, but is rather an expression of maternal responsibility. In Herland, one resident explains, "the child rearing has come to be with us a culture so profoundly studied, practiced with such subtlety and skill, that the more we love our children the less we are willing to trust that process to unskilled hands—even our own."[160] The highly engineered, scientific approach outlined in *Moving the Mountain* is adapted in *Herland* into an even more revered and "subtle" model that integrates physical education seamlessly into children's lives. Van's remark that "they had studied and overcome the 'diseases of childhood'" is quickly followed by a turn to their educational system: "they had faced the problems of education and so solved them that their children grew up as naturally as young trees."[161] He presents health and learning as closely linked and later carefully studies their early childhood education program. The Herlanders take physical education expertise to an extreme; they've "been working some sixteen hundred years, devising better and better games for children."[162] Observing the results in the "vigorous, joyous, eager little creatures" and their "steady level of good health," Van determines that physical education is central to their development.[163]

Extensions of *Moving the Mountain*'s "child gardens," *Herland*'s early childhood educational centers are designed to facilitate physical activity. "Physical properties come first" in the curriculum.[164] The facilities "had in them nothing to hurt—no stairs, no corners, no small loose objects to swallow, no fire."[165] Such a "babies' paradise," *Herland* proposes, requires a built environment that is both safe and educational.[166] The Herlander children, "taught, as rapidly as feasible, to use and control their own bodies," Van observes, are not only physically able—"sure-footed, steady-handed"—but also mentally so; they appear "clear-headed little things."[167] The centers are also engineered to encourage play. Van notes, for instance, "a sort of rubber rail raised an inch or two above the soft turf or heavy rugs" upon which toddlers practice walking.[168] "Surely we have noticed how children love to get up on something and walk along it!," he remarks of American adults. "But we have never thought to provide that simple and inexhaustible form of amusement and physical education for the young."[169] Just as Addams sought to channel adolescent desires for recreation into more wholesome activities, so too do Gilman's Herlanders apply their expertise to structure children's innate desire for physical expression.

Beyond learning about the nation's pedagogical ethos by way of observation, Van actually participates in it. Early in the novel, he and the other men with whom he is traveling are subjected to methods not unlike those he later witnesses in the child gardens. When he remarks of the training of children, "this was education for citizenship," he alludes to the fact that he himself has been put through a similar assimilation program.[170] The men are incorporated into Herland's body politic through a series of instructive activities. The novel traces Van's gradual "improvement" by portraying his adaptation to his new environment, and the text culminates with his marriage to an ideal reproductive partner: a Herlander woman. The men's education begins shortly after their arrival, when they are forcibly enrolled in an educational program designed to familiarize them with their new home. As new residents, they are immediately put in the position of pupils, and Van remarks that the "fullness of knowledge" the Herlanders exhibit "made us feel like schoolchildren."[171] The men begin studying the national language in textbooks, and it is as part of this comprehensive learning process that they participate in the country's physical culture exercises. When they take part in the Herlanders' games, Van quickly realizes their educational slant, dismissing them as "rather uninteresting" and "more like race or a—a competitive examination, than a real game with some fight in it."[172] Jeff, a doctor and, by the novel's end, the most thoroughly "Herlandized" man, disagrees: "But they are interesting—I like them . . . and I'm sure they are educational."[173] Van and Jeff's companion, Terry, however, protests that he is "sick and tired of being educated," and this refusal of their pedagogy ultimately leaves him unable to assimilate to Herland.[174]

This depiction of the men's indoctrination and assimilation reflects Gilman's concerns about national homogeneity in response to rising rates of immigration. A far cry from Addams's cosmopolitan sensibilities, Gilman was wary of the characteristics—both cultural and physiological—that immigrants brought to the United States. While Addams believed that democracy was forged by celebrating differentiation, Gilman argued that "the more kinds of races we have to reach, with all their differing cultures, ideas, tastes, and prejudices, the slower and harder is the task of developing democracy."[175] Invoking Boas's "American type," Gilman defined a "nation" as "a self-supporting group of people long enough associated in one country to form a certain type and to develop a certain culture of its own."[176] Gilman feared that the defects she perceived in poor immigrants would undermine the elevated "type" she sought. In fact, she viewed these populations less as "immigrants" than as "imported" laborers—a group in which she included "our imported millions of Africans and their descendants"—and routinely questioned their fitness for American society.[177]

Gilman delineates the threat that foreign health habits pose to the United States in *Herland*'s sequel, *With Her in Ourland* (1916), which depicts Van's global travels with his Herlander wife, Ellador. Gilman, who claimed elsewhere that "those races where the children are most absolutely subservient, as with the Chinese and Hindu . . . are not races of free and progressive thought and healthy activity," portrays Asian women in her novel as especially inept physical educators.[178] Ellador is dismayed in China to find only "crippled women" and is shocked to learn that "it is the women, their own mothers, who bind the feet of the little ones."[179] Foot binding was one of Gilman's favorite illustrations of both American supremacy and the eugenic dangers of uninformed child-rearing. In *Concerning Children*, she uses it as an example of how parental habits, rather than biology, dictate child health: "the dwindled feet of the Chinese ladies are not transmitted; but the Chinese habits [of foot binding] are."[180] Indeed, Gilman routinely held up Asian women as a eugenic threat. Later, in *With Her in Ourland*, Ellador is "eager to know about the health and physical development of the Japanese" after observing the "patient ignominy in which the women lived."[181] "How is it dear," she asks Van, "that these keenly intelligent people fail to see that such limited women cannot produce a nobler race?"[182] For Gilman, as Asha Nadkarni notes, "the downtrodden and potentially dangerous Asian woman" emerges "as eugenic feminism's foil," and this is especially true in regard to health and physical training.[183]

Motherhood is central to Ellador's views of immigration as well. Upon learning about the influx of immigrants to the United States, she responds, according to Van, "as if a mother had learned that her baby was an idiot."[184] Despite this eugenically coded critique, Ellador is convinced that the American body politic can be rehabilitated. Adopting Van's metaphor, she remarks, "the Child is by no means hopeless—in fact, I begin to think it is a very promising child."[185] In a chapter tellingly titled "The Diagnosis," she explains, "legitimate immigration is like the coming of children to you—new blood for the nation, citizens made, not born. And they should be met like children, with loving welcome, with adequate preparation, with the fullest and wisest education for their new place."[186] Ellador proposes a pedagogy of Americanization that, by infantilizing immigrants, underscores the need for maternal influence in the processes of assimilation. Though not voiced by Ellador herself, the novel also argues that such an approach has been successful in the past. When Van describes the colonization of North America to Ellador as "one of our national shames," he explains of Indigenous people, "we killed them," but reassures her by alluding to the formation of schools like Carlisle: "There has been a good deal of education and missionary work; some Indians have become fully civilized—as good citizens as any."[187] As demonstrated in the previous chapter, the education that Gilman endorses here promotes "civilization" through dangerous efforts to eradicate embodied difference.

Gilman's somewhat abstract construction of immigrants as educable children in *With Her in Ourland* is rooted in the more concrete proposal she outlined in a 1914 essay on "Immigration, Importation, and Our Fathers." She explains that "blood does not itself constitute Americanship," but rather "a national psychology is what must be shared for true citizenship."[188] Such a psychology might be instilled in European immigrants, she proposes, through a "National Training School of Citizenship" in which immigrants must enroll upon arrival.[189] In this program, she continues, "old and young, men and women, should here be trained, mentally, morally, and physically, as to health, as to clothing, as to the moral standards and manners of the country; trained in the language, history, hopes, and purposes, trained by a great corps of teachers—the best that the country could offer."[190] This hypothetical "compulsory education" is strikingly similar to the physical, mental, and moral training that Van and his companions undergo in Herland, and echoes Gilman's ongoing concerns about the role of expertise in education. In *Moving the Mountain*, too, she imagines an American future in which, with such a program of "Compulsory Socialization" and a "standard of citizenship" in place, "no immigrant is turned loose on the community til he or she is up to a certain standard, and the children we educate."[191] Gilman suggests that despite perceived corporeal differences (variations in "blood"), immigrants to the United States are, like the men in *Herland*, assimilable through physical intervention.

Her curative ideology is closely intertwined with eugenic logic. Toward the conclusion of *Herland*, the ultimately uneducable Terry attempts to sexually assault a local, demonstrating his inability to adapt to the society's moral code. Terry's transgression is presented as evidence of his biological deviance—what Gilman elsewhere called "excessive masculinity."[192] As Gail Bederman has observed, Gilman viewed sexual violence as indicative of men's evolutionary inferiority; in *Herland* his attempted rape of a citizen serves as evidence of Terry's unfitness for the society to which he has unwittingly immigrated.[193] Indeed, the indoctrinated Van, who "had learned to see these things very differently since living with Ellador," adopts a medicalized, eugenic vocabulary that differentiates Terry from his companions.[194] After the assault, "Terry dashed about like a madman" before being stopped by two Herlander women, one of whom later monitors him "as sadly patient as a mother with a degenerate child."[195] "He was crazy to be out of it all," Van continues. "It made him sick, he said, *sick*; this everlasting mother-mother-mothering. I don't think Terry had what the phrenologists call 'the lump of philoprogenitiveness' at all well developed."[196] The notion that he lacks the innate parental instinct so valorized by Herlanders codes Terry's violent behavior as a specifically eugenic defect that makes him wholly ineligible for citizenship.

This eugenic language also carries over to Gilman's imagined assimilationist programs in her essay "A Suggestion on the Negro Problem," published in the *American Journal of Sociology* in 1909. Gilman's essay expresses her fear that the majority of African Americans are "below a certain grade of citizenship" and thus "degenerating into an increasing percentage of social burdens or actual criminals."[197] Metaphorically figuring the nation as a body, Gilman explains that "the civilization of the negro" is essential to the "organic relations" of American society, as "it is quite essential to the body's life that even its least important parts be healthy."[198] She proposes the mass "enlistment" of African Americans "who are not self-supporting" (that is, poor) into a mandatory labor army—a system that she insists "is not enslavement."[199] Her vision includes enrolling children in "a system of education, the best we have," which will "guarantee the fullest development possible to each."[200] Such a program, she declares, "should furnish good physical training and as much education as each individual can take."[201] Echoing the mid-nineteenth-century racist scientific claims discussed in chapter 3 that deemed African Americans unable to care for themselves, Gilman promises that "with proper food, suitable hours of work, rest, and amusement; without the strain of personal initiative and responsibility to which so many have proved unequal," African Americans might achieve the degree of physical fitness she deems imperative to "civilization."[202]

In addition to targeting racialized groups, Gilman proposes physical training as a cure for the eugenic category with which Addams was most concerned: criminals.[203] For a 1900 article in the *Saturday Evening Post* on "Mending Morals by Making Muscles," she reflects on patients at the Elmira Reformatory, which she claims houses "hopeless criminals—absolute 'degenerates' with all their 'stigmata' upon them."[204] She reports that the patients "were submitted to the influences of the finest physical culture, to which they responded most remarkably," thus proving, in her estimate, that "the worst criminal can be sensibly improved by the best physical culture."[205] While Addams imagined physical education as a preventive health measure against criminality, Gilman sees it as a curative tool. Gilman elaborates on this further in *Moving the Mountain*, in which one character remarks, "it is really astonishing to see how much can be done with what we used to call criminals, merely by first class physical treatment," including "wonderful instruction."[206] In *Herland*, too, the men's criminalized outsider status is treated with physical education; it is in the chapter titled "A Peculiar Imprisonment" that they begin their tutelage in a Herlander culture that includes extensive exercise. Similarly, when Van asks Ellador, "Have you *no* punishments?" she replies by asking, "do you punish a person for a broken leg or a fever? We have preventive measures, and cures; sometimes we have to 'send the patient to bed,' as it were; but that's not a punishment—it's only part of the treatment."[207] By "send[ing] the patient to bed," the Herlanders attempt to make moral interventions by tending to the body. At a time when criminality was viewed as a heritable biological trait, Gilman proposes rehabilitating incarcerated people by transforming their bodies.

There is, however, a limit to Gilman's belief in human plasticity. While she imagines "improving" those marked by race and criminality, the confluence of the two appears insurmountable. In "A Suggestion on the Negro

Problem," she explains that not all African Americans are viable for a program of racial development. She clarifies that "a certain percentage of degenerates and criminals would have to be segregated and cared for" separately from the larger population.[208] She provides little elaboration on this specialized program, but claims that "the saving to the state in cutting off the supply of these degenerates would go far to establish the economy of the proposition."[209] By advocating for "cutting off the supply," Gilman couches a negative eugenics project in economic terms. She proposes that eliminating presumably dependent African Americans will save the funds necessary to implement the physical education of those she deems more "fit." Gilman's rehabilitative agenda complicates the binary of "fit" and "unfit" populations to reveal a spectrum of malleability while also adhering to eugenic determinism regarding certain populations. As Jennifer Hudak has argued, Gilman's theories represent an "uneasy negotiation" between nature and nurture.[210] Just as Margaret Fuller imagined the deterioration of Indigenous women as the grounds upon which white womanhood might flourish, Gilman positions negative eugenics as economically necessary in order to biologically improve social groups deemed redeemable.

Well before the term "fitness" was used to denote athleticism, Gilman's desire to standardize American embodiments reveals the entanglement of physical education with eugenic feminism's pursuit of homogeneity. Physical education offered a complement to selective reproduction insofar as it was a strategy for further enhancing the bodies and minds of those already deemed fit for citizenship. In "Immigration, Importation, and Our Fathers," Gilman defines "America" as "certain Ideas, Ideals, Qualities, Modes of Conduct, Institutions."[211] For Gilman, all of these were standard features that would be shared among all Americans in order to limit variation and bolster a national "type." For Addams, on the other hand, embodied American "qualities" and "modes of conduct" were inevitably varied, and it was their conglomeration that defined the changing body politic. At the same time, though, Addams saw supervised "institutions" as a means of regulating difference, ensuring that cultural and racial variations did not give way to disparities in morality. While they disagreed about the value of diversity, both Addams and Gilman ultimately relied on the expertise of white, US-born physical education experts to grapple with difference and shape the nation's citizenry.

Epilogue
From Physical Education to Wellness

In February 2020, the Mattel toy company launched its Barbie Wellness Collection, a new line of dolls promoting "meditation, physical well-being, and self-care."[1] Like all Barbies, the dolls—including Barbie Breathe with Me Doll and the Barbie Spa Doll—come with garments and accessories representative of their eponymous themes. The Barbie Fitness Doll, for instance, dons leggings and a pink tank top with "GRL PWR" emblazoned on her chest. She also comes with a set of hand weights, a gym bag, a yoga mat, a hula hoop, a water bottle, a protein bar, and a puppy. The toys' release spawned a backlash not just against the dolls themselves, but also against the contemporary culture of feminized domestic health science that has come to be known and marketed as "wellness." "Barbie Is Doing 'Self-Care' Now, and I Think We've Gone Too Far," bemoaned an article with the subheading, "Hey, kids, welcome to the wellness industry. It's expensive here."[2] The author worried that such toys risked "turning young girls into enthusiastic customers instead of healthy, well-rounded women." Another warned, "New Wellness Barbies Lead Children to the Gruesome Altar of Self-Care" and joked, "finally, a toy to teach our youth to go to $25 yoga classes, stand in line at Sweetgreen, and not ask any bigger questions about why everyone is self-soothing so very much."[3] Both the wellness Barbies themselves and the critiques of them make clear that in the twenty-first century, domestic health science has evolved into a consumer product, one insistent on selling a distorted version of empowered womanhood—GRL PWR, as it were.

Today, the domestic advice manuals and physical education advocates of the nineteenth century have given way to wellness influencers who dole out guidance on social media. Wellness, like physical education, is defined in part by its differentiation from medicine. Much like Catharine Beecher, Lydia Maria Child, and other nineteenth-century writers, wellness advocates may cite the expertise of physicians in order to legitimize their claims, but they are rarely themselves physicians.[4] Twenty-first-century wellness has converted this lay approach to health into big business. The largest sectors of the multi-trillion-dollar global wellness industry—personal care and beauty products, nutrition and food, and physical activity—typically either take place at home or in private studios rather than in clinical settings.[5] Wellness also shares nineteenth-century physical education's gendered nature. For many women, investment in these products is not only a means of self-care, but also a form of domestic health labor. If, as one venture capitalist put it, "women are often the chief medical officers of their families," then buying into wellness, like physical education before it, is a deeply feminized responsibility.[6]

The steep price tags that hang on wellness commodities from fitness studio memberships and skincare products to supplements and meditation apps is not incidental, but vital to maintaining its aspirational sheen.[7] Indeed, "aspiration"—the term that actress turned mogul Gwyneth Paltrow herself uses to describe her (in)famous lifestyle brand, Goop, has been foundational to modern wellness culture since its inception in the mid-twentieth century.[8] In his 1959 article "What High-Level Wellness Means," chief of the National Office of Vital Statistics Halbert L. Dunn explained that there was no "optimum *level* of wellness."[9] Rather, he explained, "wellness is *a direction* in progress toward an ever-higher potential of functioning."[10] This constant striving continues to define wellness culture in the twenty-first century, when, as Jia Tolentino puts it, women in particular are conditioned to "understand relentless self-improvement as natural, mandatory, and feminist—or just, without question, the best way to live."[11] Brands capitalize on and reinforce their customers' desires to better themselves physically, mentally, and spiritually, and this persistently inward gaze can redirect attention away from the tenets of a more equitably "well" society such as access to quality health care and public safety.[12] By suggesting that one's health status is a result of an individual consumer's decisions and behaviors, wellness perpetuates what Robert Crawford calls "healthism," an approach to well-being that depoliticizes health and distracts from the need to reimagine the ways that health-promoting resources are distributed.[13]

The COVID-19 pandemic has only intensified both the cultural fixation on wellness and the inequities it obscures. When municipal social distancing mandates began going into effect across the United States in March 2020, the already feminized science of wellness became further domesticated as women (and others) returned en masse to the home. As one "consumer insight strategist" put it in 2020, the "home has . . . turned into a wellness hub."[14] Some wellness "gurus" promised protections against the physical threat of the virus. In March of 2020, as lockdowns were beginning around the world, lifestyle influencer and Moon Juice founder Amanda Chantal Bacon identified herself as an "immunomodulation enthusiast" in an Instagram post prescribing "liposomal C a few times a day, high doses of D, Reishi every day, Zinc+B6, sleep, regulate cortisol (meditation + adaptogens), broth with garlic and ginger, Acupuncture, optimal magnesium levels, a cold minute to your shower."[15] Such online health advice became, in many cases, dangerous; wellness's general skepticism toward mainstream medicine quickly made it a vehicle for spreading health misinformation.[16] Even when not spreading advice for safeguarding against the virus itself, influencers portrayed social distancing as an opportunity for physical and mental personal growth. Of course, the reality was that most people who could afford to purchase expensive wellness commodities could also afford to keep themselves safe by staying isolated and working remotely or having groceries and other essentials delivered. These consumers were also statistically more likely to recover from COVID-19.[17] The health disparities highlighted by the pandemic both echo and intersect with those that the wellness industry depends on. As journalist Amy Larocca observed in early 2020, "good health has become a premium luxury product," in ways that the pandemic both exacerbated and laid bare.[18]

Like nineteenth-century physical education advocates, many wellness influencers suggest that obtaining good health is essential to leading a fulfilling, successful life. Also like physical education, wellness's model of ideal womanhood is extremely narrow. As Anna Kirkland observes, "the hallmarks of achieved wellness: slenderness, flexibility, relaxation, control, a delicate appetite—are the visage of elite female beauty in our society" and are generally associated with whiteness or an orientalist appropriation of Eastern traditions.[19] The wellness industry's insistence that it "empowers" women does little to unsettle this hegemonic model of femininity. Rather, wellness's rhetoric of empowerment insists that by becoming an ideal economic subject (that is, by purchasing wellness commodities) consumers can become an ideal woman.[20]

Wellness culture depends on its adherents' status not only as consumers but also as laborers. Beyond selling expensive products, the industry serves capitalism by striving to facilitate productivity and minimize health care costs, as the popularity of workplace wellness programs demonstrates.[21] Tolentino describes the goal of one particularly trendy exercise class as "getting you in shape for a hyperaccelerated capitalist life," revealing wellness as a health-coded version of corporate empowerment discourse.[22] In October 2022, for instance, the business publication *Forbes* published an article on "How and Why Women Can and Should Prioritize Their Wellness," in which the author reflects on how identifying what she calls "my brand of feminism" helped her realize that "women need to pursue their health more ardently and actively, maybe even more than our counterparts, as we go about the work of establishing a place for ourselves and learning to merge demanding traditional roles with additional demanding work commitments."[23] In other words, health could be the key to having it all, but only if "all" refers to corporate success, domestic normativity, and a rather stripped-down "brand of feminism" that's not so much radical as it is marketable. Indeed, mainstream wellness culture offers what Kirkland and Amanda J. Grigg describe as a "women-centered healthism that shares some features of feminism but lacks its structural critique and politicized edge."[24]

Both leading up to and during the pandemic, healthist discourse has framed the acquisition of health as individual women's private responsibility. As a result, companies sell wellness by framing it as something consumers lack. Indeed, brands often suggest that the majority of their prospective customers are currently ill. Echoing nineteenth-century writers such as Harriet Martineau's and Charlotte Perkins Gilman's insistence that American women were overwhelmingly frail, Goop's head of content, Elise Loehnen, insists that "for the most part, people are finding more and more that everyone they know is kind of sick. . . . People are self-identifying as sick much, much more."[25] Indeed, upon arriving at the In Goop Health wellness summit, the journalist Taffy Brodesser-Akner reported encountering "an autoimmune disease at every corner, be it thyroid disease, arthritis or celiac disease; trust them, you have one."[26] Goop and its competitors profit off of this ever-expanding identification with illness and subsequent desire for health. The wellness industry, as Rina Raphael notes in *The Gospel of Wellness* (2022), "is becoming almost as prescriptive as the medical industry," but its pricey solutions are not covered by health insurance, even for those who have it.[27]

Wellness companies position their protocols and products as subversive solutions and expressions of resistance to an unsatisfying medical establishment that too often neglects women's health concerns—especially those of women of color.[28] Though it purports to grant women agency over their bodies and their health, the wellness industry has commodified the feminist critique of discriminatory medicine that emerged in the mid-twentieth century through organizations such as the National Women's Health Network, the National Black Women's Health Project, and the Boston Women's Health Collective.[29] For these groups, self-care practices such as publishing accessible health information and forming discussion groups were radical responses to a medical system that failed to meet their needs.

As numerous recent articles attest, it has become nearly impossible to comment on how far mainstream self-care has strayed from these radical roots without invoking the Black feminist writer Audre Lorde.[30] In a now ubiquitous 1988 quote, Lorde insists that "caring for myself is not self-indulgence, it is self-preservation and that is an act of political warfare," launched from her multiply marginalized position while living with cancer.[31] Disability studies scholars Sami Schalk and Jina B. Kim express the importance of reclaiming "a radical politics of self-care [that] is inextricably tied to the lived experiences and temporalities of multiply marginalized people, especially disabled queer people, disabled people of color, and disabled queer people of color."[32] Despite overwhelming messaging that wellness can be bought and sold, they argue that radical self-care can and does persist outside its co-optation under capitalism.

In a world where, as Lorde put it, their communities "were never meant to survive," contemporary women writers are critiquing the mainstream wellness industry while also offering alternative models steeped in anticapitalist ideologies.[33] These writers echo those I discuss in previous chapters who adapted physical education into a political tool, and they extend the legacy of late twentieth-century activists who conceived of self-care as a mode of community endurance. As Rachel O'Neill argues, wellness is not only a luxury good—it also attracts women for whom the pursuit is "not about optimization but is instead about fortification" against the "generalized precarity" that many communities are experiencing.[34] Writers including Sonya Huber, Fariha Róisín, Jessamyn Stanley, and Tricia Hersey describe their efforts to cultivate physical and mental health outside the bounds of a largely racist, colonial, fatphobic, and ableist wellness industry. These writers refuse wellness's narrowly defined scripts while also negotiating the material necessity of self-care from their marginalized positions.

Given that its health promises presume a preexisting state of illness, it's no surprise that wellness is frequently posited as a solution for people living with chronic illnesses. Yoga in particular is recommended to people with chronic conditions so often that it has become something of an inside joke. The suggestion is ubiquitous enough that two chronically ill women chose "Have You Tried Yoga?" as the title of a podcast about managing their health.[35] Writer Sonya Huber, who lives with rheumatoid arthritis, similarly quips in *Pain Woman Takes Your Keys, and Other Essays from a Nervous System* (2017) that "the massive gulf separating the pained from the non-pained can be summed up in one question: 'Have you tried yoga?'"[36] Huber admits that she has indeed tried yoga, which she practices as one of a host of pain management techniques. Nonetheless, she finds the suggestion invalidating. "What you don't see," she imagines replying to the unsolicited advice, "is that have-you-tried-yoga is a refusal to see this massive ocean and all the million ways I have tried to swim in it."[37] As her sink-or-swim metaphor suggests, managing chronic pain makes wellness at once an urgent and a somewhat futile pursuit rather than a simple solution.

For Huber, this recurrent inquiry and those like it—"have you tried turmeric?," "have you tried meditation?," "try this cream," "buy some fish oil"— reflect a broader "reflexive need for purchased relief" that chronic conditions, by their very definition, unsettle.[38] These often expensive and quickly accumulating wellness commodities can do little to reverse her pain, and acknowledging this fact is essential to her critique. Because wellness culture cannot make her healthy, Huber sees herself as "a burr in the hide of the marketplace itself, a reminder that not all pain can be treated with a purchase."[39] Imagining her experience as a prickling "burr," Huber reroutes her pain, suggesting that it impacts not only her own body, but also a consumer culture intent on alleviating it. The persistent nature of her pain exposes the hollowness of wellness's grandiose aims.

Yoga plays an important role in Fariha Róisín's critique of mainstream wellness culture, too. She argues that reclaiming yoga and other appropriated Eastern wellness practices requires a decolonial approach steeped in historical inquiry. A South Asian woman living with irritable bowel syndrome (IBS), Róisín recalls of her early efforts to manage her condition, "so many of the practices I was gravitating toward—namely Ayurveda, meditation, and yoga—were rooted in my cultural lineage, and yet I couldn't afford access to a lot of them."[40] In *Who Is Wellness For?* (2022), Róisín describes how many such long-standing "knowledge systems" that have been repackaged by the modern wellness industry were previously "demonized, denigrated, and thwarted because they were seen as threatening to the status quo" by colonial regimes.[41] Róisín calls capitalism's obfuscation of Eastern traditions a form of "epistemicide" and calls for practitioners to revisit the histories of these practices that predate colonial frameworks. For example, she insists that "in order to meditate, you should know the history, and you should also think of why you've never had to think of this before."[42] An alternative to conventional self-help, *Who Is Wellness For?* is filled not only with self-care advice, but also with detailed accounts of both the origins of recently co-opted South Asian practices and the political histories that have obscured their origins. For instance, Róisín describes managing her IBS through an Ayurvedic protocol that she calls "my people's diet."[43] The historical relationship Róisín articulates recasts a diet that has become increasingly popular in recent years (in 2020, *Shape* magazine published the brazenly titled "Your Complete Guide to the Ayurvedic Diet," authored by a white woman and featuring an Instagram post showing two other white women laughing in a field).[44] For Róisín, however, maintaining an Ayurvedic diet is a process not only of healing her gut or achieving aestheticized wellness, but also, as she puts it, of "reclaiming my DNA."[45] The "self" that Róisín cares for is more than skin deep—it is inextricable from her history and inheritance.

Recognizing the widespread need for such reclamation, Róisín cofounded Studio Ānanda, an online resource that promotes anti-colonial approaches to wellness. At Studio Ānanda wellness entails, among other things, "global, post-capitalist healing."[46] The organization seeks to broaden both the definition of wellness and, as a result, the positionalities of those who benefit from it. Framed as a virtual "studio," the organization offers a sharp contrast to the kinds of white-owned wellness studios where Róisín had previously volunteered in exchange for free yoga classes. Its practices, too, go far beyond conventional classes. Just as *Who Is Wellness For?* narrates the historical lineages of South Asian wellness practices, part of Studio Ānanda's mission involves "archiving stories and conversations," a practice that fortifies contemporary reclamations of Indigenous wellness knowledge against further marginalization and co-optation. As both studio and archive, Studio Ānanda makes clear that historical documentation itself can be a wellness practice, one that simultaneously undermines and exposes capitalist constructions of what it means to be well.

Indeed, online tools have become just as vital to challenging the wellness industry's hegemonic standards as they are to maintaining them. Among the most prominent wellness influencers to push back on the industry's conventional standards is fat, Black, queer yoga teacher Jessamyn Stanley, who uses platforms such as Instagram (and, more recently, OnlyFans) to make space for herself and others who feel devalued by Westernized yoga's overwhelmingly thin, white aesthetic. Like Róisín, Stanley cofounded her own "inclusive digital wellness experience," "The Underbelly," as an alternative to mainstream wellness platforms.[47] Stanley argues that digital classes are instrumental in allowing yoga to become a *domestic* practice. When she first took up yoga, Stanley found that practicing at home empowered her in ways that studio classes did not. Of her early home practice, Stanley writes, "I began to see how much I restrain myself in public, making myself small and trying not to be noticed. But at home, I found myself contorting and emitting sounds I'd never had the confidence to express in public. I stopped apologizing for being loud and granted myself permission to take up space."[48]

"My yoga," she explains, is about "finding out what it means to be a Black queer woman in a world that doesn't want me to be."[49] In her first book, *Every Body Yoga: Let Go of Fear, Get on the Mat, Love Your Body* (2017), Stanley promotes a similar message, championing self-acceptance as an alternative version of wellness. In some ways, the text echoes nineteenth-century domestic health books: it contains instructive images of various exercises along with text describing their benefits. That book, she explains in the introduction, is "for every person who is self-conscious about their body."[50] Yoga, she insists, is not a method of controlling the body, but a framework for embracing it.

Just a few years later, Stanley's second book, *Yoke: My Yoga of Self-Acceptance* (2021), explores the ways in which even her own liberatory approach to yoga has been distorted by capitalism. Róisín's criticisms of the wellness industry become, in Stanley's hands, a highly self-aware reflection that reveals what happens when feminist critique becomes a wellness commodity in its own right. In one essay in *Yoke* entitled "It's a Full-Time Job Loving Yourself," she reflects on a period of weight gain that her social media followers noticed, and which, in turn, made her self-conscious of her body. The experience prompted her to realize that her own "body positivity has only ever extended as far as White supremacy will let it."[51] She notes that this experience of scrutinizing her own body in response consumers' criticisms is not a personal failing, but rather "proof that capitalism has figured out how much to monetize a commodified version of my Truth."[52]

"Self-acceptance," one of Stanley's core concepts, does not exist within a vacuum, but is shaped and, often, curtailed by the same insidious forces that necessitate it. Both images of Stanley's body and her public performances of body acceptance have become wellness commodities insofar as consuming her image on social media (and in various corporate advertisements) helps others foster self-love. Indeed, one writer describes Stanley as "*offering up herself* as evidence that true physical empowerment comes . . . from self-acceptance."[53] For Stanley, this dynamic, in which evidence that "a fat Black person can find a way to love themselves" implies that everyone should be capable of doing so, only further stigmatizes her already marginalized body.[54] Striving to imagine an alternative, she asks, "what happens when my yoga stops making thin White people feel good about themselves? . . . What happens when my body positivity stops being about them and (finally) starts being about me?"[55] Such questioning opens up the possibility of far more radical approaches to wellness that resist the instrumentalization of marginalized bodies and instead center the needs and experiences of those who live in them.

One strategy for pursuing wellness outside such capitalist imperatives might be to simply give it a rest. According to Tricia Hersey, founder of the Nap Ministry, resting is both a refusal to participate in what she identifies as the "grind culture" born of racial capitalism and a form of self and community "reverence."[56] Hersey's womanist philosophy of rest, like Róisín's decolonial approach to wellness, is grounded in history.[57] In *Rest Is Resistance: A Manifesto* (2022), she recalls developing her theology of radical rest while studying histories of anti-Black terrorism in seminary. This history, for Hersey, is personal. In *Rest Is Resistance*, she expresses her "refusal to donate my body to a system that still owes a debt to my Ancestors for the theft of their labor and DreamSpace."[58] As a Black woman in the United States, Hersey comes from what she calls "a legacy of exhaustion" that she insists must "stop with" her.[59] She recalls, for instance, how her grandmother, whom she calls her "muse," rested her eyes daily in a ritual that Hersey eventually came to recognize as a habit of routinely withdrawing from the enduring effects of the trauma of Jim Crow. She sees grind culture as a public health threat, too, citing it as a source of Black Americans' disproportionate chronic health conditions, such as her own father's ultimately fatal diabetes. Rest, for Hersey, is a protest against the harmful rhythms of racial capitalism and, as such, a form of reparations for Black Americans.

Since 2016, Hersey has hosted free Collective Napping Experiences that invite participants to rest together both virtually and in person. Such special events are not the only way to practice radical rest, though, as Hersey's manifesto makes clear. "Resting," she insists, "can look like" everything from "closing your eyes for ten minutes" or "daydreaming by staring out of a window" to "a twenty-minute timed nap" or "taking regular breaks from social media."[60] Such deliberate forms of rest, Hersey argues, don't simply repair historical injury; they enable communities to look ahead, "toward a rested future."[61] She insists that "we must imagine a new way" forward, driven by forces outside of capitalism and white supremacy and that "a slow and consistent practice" of rest is vital to enacting this radical aim.[62]

One crucial element of the "new way" Hersey champions is a transformed approach to wellness itself. Indeed, Hersey sees her work as "a total pause on everything we have ever been taught about wellness from a white supremacist, capitalist lens."[63] While Stanley laments the way her own body and her acceptance of it have been commodified through social media, Hersey is insistent that our bodies are "the only thing we own."[64] Though she promotes her work online, Hersey is wary of the way that technology and digital media usurp time that might otherwise be spent resting. She takes periodic social media "sabbaths" for months at a time and encourages others to do the same as a means of thwarting social media companies' "perfect plan to keep us distracted and addicted."[65] Hersey laments that "even those who claim to be part of the wellness industry are pushing hustling, grinding, capitalism, girl boss, competition, and coopting the work of Indigenous practices for clout and money."[66] Wary of her own practice being similarly distorted by the industry, Hersey is not interested in "connecting to our rest in a capitalist, trendy, consumer-driven way," but rather in pursuing rest as "an embodied practice and a lifelong unraveling" of the pressures of living under racial capitalism.[67] Rather than brand rest as a wellness commodity ripe for marketing, Hersey presents her work as a form of nonparticipation in a violent system of which the wellness industry is itself part.

Both the rise of the wellness industry and radical efforts to undermine it demonstrate that wellness can be an instrument of both the hegemonic and the subversive ideologies to which women subscribe. As a tool that writers employ to probe the meanings attached to gender, race, and colonialism, wellness represents the twenty-first-century expression of physical education's vexed political significance. The history I've traced throughout this book reveals that wellness, like its nineteenth-century predecessor, is a domestic health science that can be attached to a range of US feminist rhetorics. If the mainstream wellness industry represents the ongoing risks of politics predicated on a narrowly defined notion of health, writers like Huber, Róisín, Stanley, and Hersey remind us that well-being itself remains a contested concept. Taken together, their writings reveal that, far from having resolved the tensions physical education laid bare, women in the twenty-first century continue to pursue regressive and radical ends alike—all under the banner of health.

Notes

Introduction

1. *Proceedings of the Woman's Rights Convention*, 18.
2. *Proceedings of the Woman's Rights Convention*, 18.
3. *Proceedings of the Woman's Rights Convention*, 18.
4. *Proceedings of the Woman's Rights Convention*, 18.
5. On early women physicians, see Morantz-Sanchez, *Sympathy and Science*; More, Fee, and Parry, eds., *Women Physicians and the Cultures of Medicine*.
6. Phelps, *Lectures to Young Ladies*, 49.
7. Tompkins, *Racial Indigestion*, 6.
8. Rusert, *Fugitive Science*; Minich, *Radical Health*.
9. Lora Romero explains that though the ideology of domesticity can hardly be considered feminist in contemporary terms, it did provide women with a mode of "antipatriarchal analysis" and a language for describing and critiquing gender politics. See Romero, *Home Fronts*, 20.
10. I see physical education as related to but distinct from the nineteenth-century exercise movement known as "physical culture." Exercise was certainly a core component of early physical education instruction and by the end of the century became its central focus. However, while physical culture was largely a discourse of *self*-improvement, physical education asked women in particular to acquire health knowledge for the benefit of *others* as well.
11. Frances Cogan calls women who practiced physical education exemplars of "Real Womanhood," a cohort of "sensibly clad young women who would reshape the moral character of the nation." While Cogan suggests that this model of femininity provided a safe middle ground between the debilitating "Cult of True Womanhood" and more radical politics, I propose that such an investment in health had profound political and social reverberations. Cogan, *All-American Girl*, 61. On the "tomboy" as related model of female identity, see Abate, *Tomboys*. For more on the relationship between bodily plasticity and "character" more broadly, see Salazar, *Bodies of Reform*.
12. Tompkins, *Racial Indigestion*, 6.
13. Morantz, "Making Women Modern," 494.
14. Beecher, *Suggestions Respecting Improvements in Education*, 7.
15. Beecher, *Suggestions Respecting Improvements in Education*, 8.
16. Child, *The Mother's Book*, 58.
17. On the importance of physical education to women's higher education, see Todd, *Physical Culture and the Body Beautiful*.
18. Todd, *Physical Culture and the Body Beautiful*, 20.

19. *A Course of Calisthenics*, 1. My emphasis.

20. See Horowitz, *Rereading Sex*, 109–11; Haynes, *Riotous Flesh*, 81–106.

21. Nichols, *Lectures to Women on Anatomy and Physiology*, 17.

22. Kaplan, "Manifest Domesticity." See also Davidson and Hatcher, eds., *No More Separate Spheres!*

23. Sedgwick, *Means and Ends*, 38.

24. Sedgwick, *Means and Ends*, 271, 270.

25. Kerber, "The Republican Mother."

26. Todd, *Physical Culture and the Body Beautiful*, 221.

27. Alcott, *Little Men*, 136.

28. Vertinsky, *The Eternally Wounded Woman*.

29. Verbrugge, *Active Bodies*.

30. Verbrugge, *Active Bodies*.

31. Park, "'Embodied Selves,'" 1509.

32. Vertinsky, *The Eternally Wounded Woman*, 4.

33. Vertinsky, *The Eternally Wounded Woman*, 15.

34. Todd, *Physical Culture and the Body Beautiful*, 7. This view of nineteenth-century women mirrors feminist journalist Gloria Steinem's speculation in 1995 that "an increase in our physical strength could have more impact on the everyday lives of most women than the occasional role model in the boardroom or in the White House." Steinem, *Moving beyond Words*, 97.

35. Verbrugge, *Active Bodies*, 10.

36. Verbrugge, *Active Bodies*, 10.

37. Purkiss, *Fit Citizens*, 59–65, 170.

38. Burbick, *Healing the Republic*, 3.

39. Metzl, "Why against Health?," 2.

40. Sánchez-Eppler, *Touching Liberty*; Garland-Thomson, *Extraordinary Bodies*.

41. Baynton, "Slaves, Immigrants, and Suffragists," 562–67; Pitts, "Disability, Scientific Authority, and Women's Political Participation."

42. Seitler, *Atavistic Tendencies*; Lamp and Cleigh, "A Heritage of Ableist Rhetoric"; Nadkarni, *Eugenic Feminism*; Hayden, *Evolutionary Rhetoric*.

43. Schuller, *The Biopolitics of Feeling*.

44. Garland-Thomson, "Misfits"; Puar, *The Right to Maim*, xiv.

45. Schalk and Kim, "Integrating Race," 43.

46. Wendell, *The Rejected Body*, 93.

47. For analyses of ableist metaphors in contemporary feminist theory, see May and Ferri, "Fixated on Ability"; Schalk, "Metaphorically Speaking."

48. Elman, "Slothful Movements."

49. Doty, *The Perfecting of Nature*.

50. On the mutually influential relationship between literature and reform movements and institutions at the end of the nineteenth century especially, see Fisher, *Reading for Reform*.

51. Jacobs, *Incidents in the Life of a Slave Girl*, 276.

52. Lorde, *A Burst of Light*, 130.

Chapter One

1. Willard, *A Plan for Improving Female Education*, 13. Though the state legislature ultimately rejected her proposal, the city of Troy, New York, raised funds that allowed Willard to open the Troy Female Seminary in 1821.

2. Willard, *A Plan for Improving Female Education*, 22, 13.

3. Willard, *A Plan for Improving Female Education*, 34.

4. Willard, *A Plan for Improving Female Education*, 34.

5. Willard, *A Plan for Improving Female Education*, 34, 35.

6. Willard, *A Plan for Improving Female Education*, 35.

7. Edelstein, "Reading Age beyond Childhood," 125. See also Edelstein, *Adulthood and Other Fictions*.

8. Edelstein, *Adulthood and Other Fictions*, 19–20.

9. Edelstein, *Adulthood and Other Fictions*, 20–21; on the "Young America" literary movement as well as its political counterpart, see Wallach, *Obedient Sons*; Widmer, *Young America*, 5.

10. Harper, *Solitary Travelers*, 14.

11. Vetter, *The Political Thought of America's Founding Feminists*, 39, 35.

12. Cooper, *Correspondence of James Fenimore-Cooper*, vol. 1, 151.

13. Bederman, "Revisiting Nashoba," 438.

14. See, for example, Oravec, "Fanny Wright and the Enforcing of Prudence"; Ginzberg, "'The Hearts of Your Readers Will Shudder'"; Jackson, *American Radicals*; Kissel, *In Common Cause*; Bartlett, *Liberty, Equality, Sorority*; Deák, *Passage to America*.

15. In addition to the works by Harriet Martineau and Margaret Fuller discussed elsewhere in this chapter, such texts include English writer Frances Milton Trollope's *Domestic Manners of the Americans* (1832), which directly contradicts Wright's optimism; Caroline Kirkland's *A New Home—Who'll Follow? or, Glimpses of Western Life* (1839), which describes her life upon relocating to eastern Michigan; and Lydia Maria Child's *Letters from New-York* (1841), which she published shortly after moving to the city to edit the *National Anti-Slavery Standard*.

16. Wright, *Views of Society and Manners in America*, 82.

17. Locke, *Some Thoughts Concerning Education*, 1; Wright, *Views of Society and Manners in America*, 426.

18. Rendell, "Prospects of the American Republic, 145.

19. Rendell, "Prospects of the American Republic," 147.

20. Murison, "The Tyranny of Sleep," 247.

21. Rendell, "Prospects of the American Republic," 154.

22. Wright, *Views of Society and Manners in America*, 82.

23. Bederman, "Revisiting Neshoba," 440.

24. Altschuler, *The Medical Imagination*, 24.

25. Murison, "The Tyranny of Sleep," 253.

26. Wright, *Views of Society and Manners in America*, 453.

27. Wright, *Views of Society and Manners in America*, 453–54.

28. Wright, *Views of Society and Manners in America*, 191.

29. Wright, *Views of Society and Manners in America*, 190–91, 188.
30. Wright, *Views of Society and Manners in America*, 428.
31. Wright, *Views of Society and Manners in America*, 427.
32. Wright, *Views of Society and Manners in America*, 426.
33. Quoted in Wright, *Views of Society and Manners in America*, 34–35.
34. Wright, *Views of Society and Manners in America*, 35. Emphasis is original.
35. Quoted in Wright, *Views of Society and Manners in America*, 35.
36. Wright, *Views of Society and Manners in America*, 426.
37. Wright, *Views of Society and Manners in America*, 430.
38. Wright, *Views of Society and Manners in America*, 430.
39. Wollstonecraft, *A Vindication of the Rights of Woman*, 106–7.
40. Vetter, *The Political Thought of America's Founding Feminists*, 46.
41. Wright, *Views of Society and Manners in America*, 428, 421.
42. Wright, *Views of Society and Manners in America*, 429.
43. Wright, *Views of Society and Manners in America*, 35.
44. Kerber, "The Republican Mother."
45. Rush, *A Plan for the Establishment of Public Schools*, 34.
46. Wright, *Views of Society and Manners in America*, 421.
47. Wright, *Views of Society and Manners in America*, 430.
48. Wright, *Views of Society and Manners in America*, 428.
49. Wright, *A Lecture on Existing Evils and Their Remedy*, 7.
50. Wright, *A Lecture on Existing Evils and Their Remedy*, 7.
51. Owen and Wright, *Tracts on Republican Government and National Education*, 13; Wright, *A Lecture on Existing Evils and Their Remedy*, 7.
52. For a thorough account of Martineau's career, see Roberts, *The Woman and the Hour*.
53. Malthus, *An Essay on the Principle of Population*, 54.
54. Malthus, *An Essay on the Principle of Population*, 19.
55. Martineau, *Society in America*, vol. 2, 77.
56. Martineau, *Society in America*, vol. 2, 269.
57. Hovet, "Harriet Martineau's Exceptional American Narratives," 72.
58. For comparisons to Tocqueville, see Hovet, "Harriet Martineau's Exceptional American Narratives"; Vetter, *The Political Thought of America's Founding Feminists*. On Martineau and Trollope, see Harper, *Solitary Travelers*, 111–14. For a comparative study of Wright and Trollope, see Kissel, *In Common Cause*. Martineau later focused on health and illness more explicitly in her 1844 work *Life in the Sick-Room*.
59. Scholl, "Mediation and Expansion," 822.
60. Martineau, *Society in America*, vol. 2, 226.
61. Martineau, *Society in America*, vol. 2, 226.
62. Harriet Martineau, "On Female Education," *Monthly Repository*, February 1823, 77.
63. Martineau, "On Female Education," 78.
64. Martineau, "On Female Education," 78.
65. Wright, *Views of Society and Manners in America*, 421; Martineau, *Society in America*, vol. 2, 228.

66. Martineau, *Society in America*, vol. 2, 228.
67. Martineau, *Society in America*, vol. 2, 262.
68. Martineau, *Society in America*, vol. 2, 262.
69. Martineau, *Society in America*, vol. 2, 262.
70. Martineau, *Society in America*, vol. 2, 264.
71. Martineau, *Society in America*, vol. 2, 263.
72. Martineau, *Society in America*, vol. 2, 263.
73. Martineau, *Society in America*, vol. 2, 263–64.
74. Martineau, *Society in America*, vol. 2, 264.
75. Martineau, *Society in America*, vol. 2, 262; vol. 1, 197.
76. Martineau, *How to Observe*, 140–41.
77. Martineau, *Society in America*, vol. 2, 232, 233, 239.
78. Martineau, *Society in America*, vol. 2, 230.
79. Martineau, *Society in America*, vol. 2, 235.
80. Martineau, *Society in America*, vol. 2, 369.
81. Martineau, *Society in America*, vol. 2, 230.
82. Martineau, *Society in America*, vol. 2, 232.
83. Martineau, *Society in America*, vol. 2, 232.
84. Martineau, *Society in America*, vol. 2, 232–33.
85. Martineau, *Society in America*, vol. 2, 233.
86. Martineau, *Society in America*, vol. 2, 233.
87. Martineau, *How to Observe*, 142.
88. Martineau, *Society in America*, vol. 2, 261.
89. Martineau, *Society in America*, vol. 2, 263.
90. Martineau, *Society in America*, vol. 1, 197.
91. Martineau, *Society in America*, vol. 2, 261; vol. 1, 197.
92. Martineau, *Society in America*, vol. 2, 261; vol. 1, 197.
93. Martineau, *Society in America*, vol. 2, 261.
94. Martineau, *Society in America*, vol. 2, 345.
95. Martineau, *Society in America*, vol. 2, 345.
96. Goodlad, "Imperial Woman," 201.
97. Martineau, *Society in America*, vol. 2, 235.
98. Martineau, *Society in America*, vol. 2, 51.
99. Martineau, *Society in America*, vol. 2, 53.
100. Martineau, *Society in America*, vol. 2, 367.
101. Martineau, *Harriet Martineau's Autobiography*, vol. 2, 70.
102. Martineau, *Harriet Martineau's Autobiography*, vol. 2, 71.
103. Martineau, *Harriet Martineau's Autobiography*, vol. 2, 73.
104. Martineau, *Harriet Martineau's Autobiography*, vol. 2, 72.
105. Fuller quoted in Capper, *Margaret Fuller*, vol. 1, 155.
106. In *Woman in the Nineteenth Century*, Fuller praises Sedgwick's instructive manual, *Means and Ends*, which claims that women's "moral and intellectual" development "depend mainly" on their "physical being" (38). Fuller also favorably reviewed Catharine Beecher's writing in the *Tribune*. See Fuller, *Woman in the Nineteenth Century*, 150; Fuller, "The Wrongs of American Women."

107. For accounts of how Fuller's foray into journalism transformed her transcendentalism, see Steele, "Sentimental Transcendentalism and Political Affect," 207–8; Belasco, "'The Animating Influences of Discord,'" 76–79.

108. Hurst, "Bodies in Transition," 12. For an overview of the various attitudes toward physical education expressed by Fuller's transcendentalist peers, including Ralph Waldo Emerson, Henry David Thoreau, William Ellery Channing, and Amos Bronson Alcott, see Park, "The Attitudes of Leading New England Transcendentalists."

109. Fuller, *Woman in the Nineteenth Century*, 150.

110. Roberson, "Geographies of Expansion," 118.

111. Martineau, *Society in America*, vol. 2, 278.

112. Alcott, *Observations on the Principles and Methods of Infant Instruction*, 4; Fuller, "Autobiographical Romance," 37.

113. Quoted in Emerson, Channing, and Clarke, eds., *Memoirs of Margaret Fuller Ossoli*, vol. 1, 172.

114. Thoreau, quoted in Davis, "Margaret Fuller, Body and Soul," 34.

115. Fuller, "Autobiographical Romance," 37; Fuller, *The Letters of Margaret Fuller*, 300.

116. Fuller, *Woman in the Nineteenth Century*, 149; Locke, *Some Thoughts Concerning Education*, 2.

117. Rousseau, *Émile, or On Education*, 211.

118. Fuller, "Autobiographical Romance," 26.

119. Fuller, *Woman in the Nineteenth Century*, 27.

120. Fuller, "Autobiographical Romance," 26.

121. Fuller, "Autobiographical Romance," 26.

122. Fuller, "Autobiographical Romance," 37.

123. Fuller, "Autobiographical Romance," 27.

124. Fuller, "Autobiographical Romance," 26.

125. Fuller, "Autobiographical Romance," 27; Fuller, *Woman in the Nineteenth Century*, 149.

126. Fuller, "Physical Education," 193.

127. Fuller, *Summer on the Lakes*, 47.

128. Thoreau, "Walking," 268.

129. Valenčius, *The Health of the Country*, 11–12.

130. Wright, *Views of Society and Manners in America*, 190.

131. Wright, *Views of Society and Manners in America*, 16.

132. Wright, *Views of Society and Manners in America*, 190.

133. Wright, *Views of Society and Manners in America*, 190, 191.

134. Martineau, *Society in America*, vol. 1, 232, 264. The other healthy locales Martineau names are "the elevated parts of the Alleghany range" and "Charleston."

135. Fuller, *Summer on the Lakes*, 61.

136. Fuller, *Summer on the Lakes*, 62.

137. Fuller, *Summer on the Lakes*, 62.

138. Fish, *Black and White Women's Travel Narratives*, 121.

139. Fuller, *Woman in the Nineteenth Century*, 83.

140. Fuller, *Summer on the Lakes*, 62.

141. Fuller, *Woman in the Nineteenth Century*, 83.

142. Fuller, *Summer on the Lakes*, 63.
143. Fuller, *Summer on the Lakes*, 62.
144. Fuller, *Summer on the Lakes*, 62.
145. Thoreau, "Walden," 213. For more on Thoreau's view of nature as therapeutic, see Burbick, *Healing the Republic*; Branch and Pierce, "'Another Name for Health'"; Reiss, "Sleeping at Walden Pond."
146. Kafer, *Feminist, Queer, Crip*, 135.
147. Emerson, "The American Scholar," 57.
148. Emerson, "Nature," 29.
149. Fuller, *Summer on the Lakes*, 62.
150. Martineau, *Society in America*, vol. 1, 282.
151. Burch, *Committed*, 10; Cowing, "Occupied Land Is an Access Issue."
152. Sorisio, *Fleshing Out America*, 145–46.
153. Fuller, *Summer on the Lakes*, 173.
154. Fuller, *Woman in the Nineteenth Century*, 161, 73.
155. Fuller, *Summer on the Lakes*, 169, 179.
156. Teuton, "Disability in Indigenous North America," 573, 574.
157. Fuller, *Summer on the Lakes*, 175.
158. Kolodny, *The Land before Her*, 126.
159. Fuller, *Woman in the Nineteenth Century*, 24.
160. Fuller, *Summer on the Lakes*, 251.
161. Fuller, *Summer on the Lakes*, 251.
162. Fuller, *Summer on the Lakes*, 63.
163. Alaimo, *Undomesticated Ground*, 37.
164. Gilmore, "Margaret Fuller 'Receiving' the Indians," 193.
165. Fuller, *Summer on the Lakes*, 173.

Chapter Two

1. According to Fuller's friend and biographer Thomas Wentworth Higginson, Farrar "perceived the defects of [Fuller's] training" in the 1820s and "undertook to mould her externally." It is likely that much of the advice in Farrar's manual was similar to that which she offered the young Fuller. Higginson, *Margaret Fuller Ossoli*, 36.
2. Farrar, *The Young Lady's Friend*, 249–50.
3. Dudden, *Serving Women*, 194.
4. Sánchez-Eppler, *Dependent States*; Levander, *Cradle of Liberty*; Wright, *Black Girlhood in the Nineteenth Century*; Bernstein, *Racial Innocence*. For a related argument that focuses on the late eighteenth century, see Duane, *Suffering Childhood in Early America*.
5. Glenn, *Forced to Care*, 7.
6. Dudden, *Serving Women*, 1; Manion, *Liberty's Prisoners*, 117.
7. Kaplan, "Manifest Domesticity."
8. Baym, *Woman's Fiction*, 27.
9. Beecher, *A Treatise on Domestic Economy*, 206–7.
10. Beecher, *A Treatise on Domestic Economy*, 207.

11. Beecher, *A Treatise on Domestic Economy*, 207, 211.

12. As Nicole Tonkovich argues, Beecher and many of her contemporaries rhetorically constructed and aligned themselves with an ideal middle-class white housewife while also forging a distance between writers and servants. Tonkovich, *Domesticity with a Difference*, 128.

13. Beecher, *Letters to Persons Who Are Engaged in Domestic Service*, 127.

14. Beecher, *Letters to Persons Who Are Engaged in Domestic Service*, 126–27.

15. Beecher, *Letters to Persons Who Are Engaged in Domestic Service*, 127.

16. Beecher, *Letters to Persons Who Are Engaged in Domestic Service*, 62.

17. Beecher, *Letters to Persons Who Are Engaged in Domestic Service*, 126.

18. Beecher, *Letters to Persons Who Are Engaged in Domestic Service*, 128.

19. Beecher, *Letters to Persons Who Are Engaged in Domestic Service*, 126.

20. Beecher, *Letters to Persons Who Are Engaged in Domestic Service*, 74.

21. Beecher, *Letters to Persons Who Are Engaged in Domestic Service*, 78.

22. Dudden, *Serving Women*, 194.

23. Beecher, *Letters to Persons Who Are Engaged in Domestic Service*, 10. Anxieties about "faithful" domestic workers were rampant in the antebellum United States, as middle-class families sought household employees who would demonstrate their loyalty through both diligent labor and a lengthy (perhaps permanent) tenure. Organizations such as the Society for the Encouragement of Faithful Domestics (founded in New York) and the Philadelphia Society for the Encouragement of Faithful Domestics emerged in the 1820s as placement agencies and surveillance mechanisms that intended to provide employers with well-recommended domestics certified with "a certificate of . . . health" and simultaneously maintained a list of those deemed "unworthy" of service. Manion, *Liberty's Prisoners*, 116–17; Society for the Encouragement of Faithful Domestic Servants of New York, *First Annual Report*, 34, 7.

24. Kaplan has shown that Beecher imagined a "sovereign mother" overseeing the home by employing the language of empire ("Manifest Domesticity," 589). On the tension between the "domestic sovereignty" Beecher revered and American democracy, see Logan, *Awkward Rituals*, 108–10.

25. Beecher, *A Treatise on Domestic Economy*, 41.

26. Urban, *Brokering Servitude*, 16–17.

27. Phillips-Cunningham, *Putting Their Hands on Race*.

28. Beecher, *A Treatise on Domestic Economy*, 39.

29. Beecher, *A Treatise on Domestic Economy*, 64. Emphasis is original.

30. Beecher, *A Treatise on Domestic Economy*, 39.

31. Beecher, *A Treatise on Domestic Economy*, 213.

32. Ware, quoted in Robbins, "Periodizing Authorship, Characterizing Genre," 6. The other novels in this series are *Home* (1835) and *The Poor Rich Man, and the Rich Poor Man* (1836).

33. As Joe Shapiro notes, this view of employers as mothers reflects Sedgwick's broader endorsement of economic paternalism as an alternative to class conflict. Shapiro, *The Illiberal Imagination*, 115.

34. Sedgwick quoted in Robbins, "Periodizing Authorship, Characterizing Genre," 6. As Laurie Ousley observes, the novel is not a critique of capitalism itself, but rather

a sentimental critique of working conditions and class relations. Ousley, "The Business of Housekeeping," 137.

35. The novel's call for middle-class women to reform their treatment of domestics received a range of responses when it was published in 1837. While Reverend William Ellery Channing was pleased that "thousands, as they read it, will feel their deficiencies, and resolve to do better," a writer for the *New York Review* feared such awareness of middle-class women's failings would empower workers to a dangerous degree. "It is precisely the book," the reviewer wrote, "that we should wish to keep out of the hands of a numerous class of servants." See Sedgwick, *Life and Letters of Catharine M. Sedgwick*, 270; Baym, *Novels, Readers, and Reviewers*, 47.

36. Ryan, *Love, Wages, Slavery*, 42.
37. Sedgwick, *Live and Let Live*, 74–75.
38. Sedgwick, *Live and Let Live*, 54.
39. Sedgwick, *Live and Let Live*, 22, 21.
40. Sedgwick, *Live and Let Live*, 18.
41. Sedgwick, *Live and Let Live*, 204.
42. Sedgwick, *Live and Let Live*, 45–46.
43. Sedgwick, *Live and Let Live*, 99.
44. Sedgwick, *Live and Let Live*, 116.
45. Sedgwick, *Live and Let Live*, 116.
46. Sedgwick, *Live and Let Live*, 116, 120.
47. Sedgwick, *Live and Let Live*, 116.
48. Sedgwick, *Live and Let Live*, 78.
49. Sedgwick, *Live and Let Live*, v.
50. Sedgwick, *Live and Let Live*, 72.
51. Sedgwick, *Live and Let Live*, 17.
52. Sedgwick, *Live and Let Live*, 21.
53. Sedgwick, *Live and Let Live*, 201–2.
54. Sedgwick, *Live and Let Live*, 185.
55. Sedgwick, *Live and Let Live*, 214.
56. Sedgwick, *Live and Let Live*, 32.
57. Sedgwick, *Live and Let Live*, 32.
58. Sedgwick, *Live and Let Live*, 33.
59. Sedgwick, *Life and Letters of Catharine M. Sedgwick*, 20. Emphasis is mine.
60. Sedgwick, *Live and Let Live*, 33. When Mrs. Broadson hires Lucy in Judy's stead, she tells Bridget, "it's natural, you know, I should prefer an American girl" (33).
61. Sedgwick, *Live and Let Live*, 58, 59.
62. Palumbo-DeSimone, "'Kitchen Queens' and 'Tributary Housekeepers'"; Murphy, "The Irish Servant Girl in Literature."
63. Sedgwick, *Life and Letters of Catharine M. Sedgwick*, 21.
64. Sedgwick, *Live and Let Live*, 79.
65. Sedgwick, *Live and Let Live*, 58.
66. Sedgwick, *Live and Let Live*, 58.
67. Sedgwick, *Live and Let Live*, 79.
68. Sedgwick, *Live and Let Live*, 63.

69. Sedgwick, *Live and Let Live*, 60.
70. Sedgwick, *Live and Let Live*, 60.
71. Sedgwick, *Live and Let Live*, 59.
72. Sedgwick, *Live and Let Live*, 60.
73. Sedgwick, *Live and Let Live*, 71. Emphasis is original.
74. Sedgwick, *Live and Let Live*, 71.
75. Sedgwick, *Live and Let Live*, 91.
76. Sedgwick, *Live and Let Live*, 57.
77. Sedgwick, *Live and Let Live*, 58.
78. Sedgwick, *Live and Let Live*, 65.
79. Sedgwick, *Live and Let Live*, vi. Emphasis is original.
80. Sedgwick, *Life and Letters of Catharine M. Sedgwick*, 22.
81. Sedgwick, *Live and Let Live*, 71.
82. White, "'Our Nig' and the She-Devil."
83. Bernstein, *Racial Innocence*, 8; Wright, *Black Girlhood in the Nineteenth Century*, 61.
84. Scholars have rightly questioned the novel's place within the sentimental tradition. Julia Stern, for instance, invites us to view the novel in relation to other genres that similarly center violence against the protagonist, such as the gothic novel and the captivity narrative. Building on Stern's reading, Kyla Wazana Tompkins calls the novel an "antisentimental text" insofar as it inverts the domestic tropes of works like *Uncle Tom's Cabin*. Finally, building on work by Karsten Pier, Sam Plasencia argues that Wilson performs "postsentimental work" by foregrounding the violators rather than the victims in her depictions. Stern, "Excavating Genre in *Our Nig*"; Tompkins, *Racial Indigestion*, 118; Piep, "'Nothing New under the Sun'"; Plasencia, "Staging Enfleshment," 192–93.
85. Wilson, *Our Nig*, 4. Cynthia J. Davis suggests that her repeated references to Frado's physical injuries enables Wilson to establish Black female embodiment outside of their hypersexualization by using "pain in her narrative as a metonym for sexual exploitation." Nazera Sadiq Wright more directly addresses the loss of innocence implied by that sexualization when she argues that "the pain and suffering Frado endures and the scars on her body are intended to distance the black girl further from the white household by removing all traces of innocence from her abused body." Davis, "Speaking the Body's Pain," 398; Wright, *Black Girlhood in the Nineteenth Century*, 82.
86. Ryan makes a similar observation when she notes that "Wilson affirms much of the advice found in *Home* and *Live and Let Live* when she finds Frado's employers failing to provide a family-like work environment, to offer family-like nurture and affective sustenance to a live-in servant, and, worst of all, to extend family-like concern to a 'bound' girl who becomes ill through overwork." Ryan's focus, however, is exclusively on the employer/employee relationship, while I argue that the novel situates these within Frado's experiences with her biological mother and, later, her own child. Ryan, *Love, Wages, Slavery*, 127.
87. Tate, *Black Women Writers at Work*; Sánchez-Eppler, *Dependent States*; Lott, "Unweepable Wounds Unwept."
88. Sánchez-Eppler, *Dependent States*, 49.
89. Short, "Harriet Wilson's Our Nig and the Labor of Citizenship," 2.

90. Wilson, *Our Nig*, 9. According to Dudden, "laundry work was the most onerous part of housework, and housekeepers were eager to delegate it to a domestic or a laundress." Dudden, *Serving Women*, 143.

91. Wilson, *Our Nig*, 5.

92. Wilson's own mother, also named Margaret Smith (despite Wilson's use of pseudonyms for many other characters in her text) was similarly racialized. On March 27, 1830, the local newspaper *The Farmer's Cabinet* ran an obituary identifying her as "Margaret Ann Smith, black, late of Portsmouth, N.H." Quoted in Foreman, "Introduction" to *Our Nig*, 89. On how such kinship relationships such as Mag shared with Frado's Black father and, later, Black stepfather can transmit race and challenge genealogical notions of racial inheritances, see Fielder, *Relative Races*.

93. The anonymously authored 1855 advice book *Plain Talk and Friendly Advice to Domestics: With Counsel on Home Matters* actually uses *both* Bridget and Margaret as stand-ins for the masses of Irish women working as domestics. In Wilson's novel, Mag is not only likened to immigrant women, but actually positioned beneath them. She marries Jim at least partly out of economic necessity—her laundering work dwindles when "foreigners who cheapened toil and clamored for a livelihood," competed with her, and she could not thus sustain herself. Though seemingly separate from these "foreigners," Mag nonetheless embodies a liminal racial identity that evokes the status of many European immigrant domestics. Furthermore, in addition to signaling anti-Black racism, the novel's title, *Our Nig*, might further connect Mag's (and Frado's) plight to that of Irish immigrant women. In addition to being short for Margaret, "Mag" is also a version of the Irish surname preface, "Mac," and "Nig" an equivalent substitute for the preface, "Nic." *Plain Talk and Friendly Advice to Domestics*, 67–78.

94. Wilson, *Our Nig*, 11.

95. Wilson, *Our Nig*, 9.

96. Sedgwick, *Live and Let Live*, 71. Emphasis is original.

97. Scholars including Sally Gomaa have shown how Frado's eventual abandonment by her lover as an adult also echoes Mag's early seduction and subsequent social ruin. Gomaa, "Writing to 'Virtuous' and 'Gentle' Readers."

98. On the possibility that "Margaret Thorn" and the author of the other appended letter, "Allida" are Wilson's own narrative constructions, see Breau, "Identifying Satire," 457–58.

99. Wilson, *Our Nig*, 139. Emphasis is original.

100. Lott posits that Mag's exchange of her daughter for her own economic relief constitutes a "maternal passage" into bondage that parallels the Middle Passage across the Atlantic. Mag's adoption of Frado's stepfather's surname, "Shipley," further characterizes Mag as a vessel delivering Frado to her captivity among the Bellmonts. Lott, "Unweepable Wounds Unwept," 489.

101. Wilson, *Our Nig*, 46.

102. Wilson, *Our Nig*, 30.

103. Wilson, *Our Nig*, 139.

104. Wilson, *Our Nig*, 18.

105. Wilson, *Our Nig*, 26.

106. Wilson, *Our Nig*, 29.

107. Wilson, *Our Nig*, 29. Emphasis is original.
108. Wilson, *Our Nig*, 66. Emphasis is original.
109. Wilson, *Our Nig*, 62.
110. Leveen, "Dwelling in the House of Oppression," 567.
111. Wilson, *Our Nig*, 63.
112. Wilson, *Our Nig*, 64.
113. Wilson, *Our Nig*, 66.
114. Wilson, *Our Nig*, 109.
115. Foreman, *Activist Sentiments*, 55; Singley, "Servitude and Homelessness," 10.
116. Dudden, *Serving Women*, 22.
117. Donkor, "Laboring Bodies," 56.
118. Wilson, *Our Nig*, 30, 29.
119. Wilson, *Our Nig*, 63.
120. Wilson, *Our Nig*, 44.
121. Wilson, *Our Nig*, 29, 52.
122. Wilson, *Our Nig*, 118.
123. Wilson, *Our Nig*, 88–89.
124. Morgan, *Laboring Women*.
125. Smith, *Natural History of the Human Species*, 226.
126. Bernstein, *Racial Innocence*, 28.
127. Wilson, *Our Nig*, 66.
128. Wilson, *Our Nig*, 81–82.
129. Wilson, *Our Nig*, 120.
130. Wilson, *Our Nig*, 81.
131. Wilson, *Our Nig*, 76.
132. Lovell, "By Dint of Labor and Economy," 21.
133. Wilson, *Our Nig*, 117.
134. Wilson, *Our Nig*, 117.
135. Wilson, *Our Nig*, 120.
136. Wilson, *Our Nig*, 121.
137. Wilson, *Our Nig*, 133.
138. Wilson, *Our Nig*, 133.
139. Wilson, *Our Nig*, 4.
140. Wilson, *Our Nig*, 128. Wilson's description of Samuel's travels as "desertion" also recalls her earlier reference to Frado's "desertion by her mother" (24).
141. Wilson, *Our Nig*, 136.
142. Wilson, *Our Nig*, 139.
143. Wilson, *Our Nig*, 139.

Chapter Three

1. Lydia Maria Child, "A, B, C of Abolition: For Those Who Have Not Yet Examined the Subject; Anti-Slavery Catechism," *National Anti-Slavery Standard*, September 23, 1841.
2. "Selections," *National Anti-Slavery Standard*, May 4, 1843.

3. "Runaway Slaves," *North Star*, February 25, 1848.

4. "They Cannot Take Care of 'Themselves,'" *National Anti-Slavery Standard*, February 10, 1842.

5. Jacobs, *Incidents in the Life of a Slave Girl*, 276.

6. Jacobs, *Incidents in the Life of a Slave Girl*, 43. This passage is also reprinted, with slight changes, in "The Good Grandmother" in Child, *The Freedmen's Book*. On Child's rhetorical investments in Jacobs's account of her grandmother, see Mills, "Lydia Maria Child and the Endings."

7. Mitchell, *From Slave Cabins to the White House*, 41.

8. Following Andrea Stone, I understand "health and well-being as connected categories, the former more directly concerned with positive physical and mental experiences, which may derive from a healthful diet, exercise, and relations with others, and the latter an extension of these resources to an overall sense of happiness, energy, and fulfillment." Stone, *Black Well-Being*, 3.

9. Roberts, *Killing the Black Body*, 55.

10. Wallace-Sanders, *Mammy*.

11. In a footnote, Child writes, "The poison of a snake is a powerful acid, and is counteracted by powerful alkalies [sic], such as potash, ammonia, &c. The Indians are accustomed to apply wet ashes, or plunge the limb into strong lie. White men, employed to lay out railroads in snaky places, often carry ammonia with them as an antidote.—editor." Quoted in Jacobs, *Incidents in the Life of a Slave Girl*, 151.

12. See Beecher and Stowe, *The American Woman's Home*.

13. In *Incidents in the Life of a Slave Girl*, Jacobs recalls that her brother "thought of opening an anti-slavery reading room in Rochester, and combining with it the sale of some books and stationery; and he wanted me to unite with him. We tried it, but it was not successful. We found warm anti-slavery friends there, but the feeling was not general enough to support such an establishment." Jacobs, *Incidents in the Life of a Slave Girl*, 284.

14. Rusert, *Fugitive Science*, 4.

15. Rusert, *Fugitive Science*, 17.

16. On slavery and medical abuse in *Incidents in the Life of a Slave Girl*, see Titus, "'This Poisonous System'"; Carolyn Sorisio, *Fleshing Out America*; Berry, "'[No] Doctor but My Master.'" On the medical treatment of enslaved women more broadly, see Schwartz, *Birthing a Slave*; Washington, *Medical Apartheid*; Weiner and Hough, *Sex, Sickness, and Slavery*; Dudley, "Toward an Understanding of the 'Medical Plantation'"; Cooper Owens, *Medical Bondage*.

17. Barclay, *The Mark of Slavery*, 97–106.

18. On Cartwright's theories of sleep regulation, see Reiss, *Wild Nights*.

19. Cartwright's theories received much attention in the *Standard* in the 1850s. See, for example, "Pro-Slavery," *National Anti-Slavery Standard*, August 28, 1851; "Our Philadelphia Correspondence," *National Anti-Slavery Standard*, October 21, 1854; as well as Lydia Maria Child, "The Stars and Stripes," *National Anti-Slavery Standard*, January 30, 1858.

20. "Selections," *National Anti-Slavery Standard*, March 17, 1853.

21. Nott and Gliddon, *Types of Mankind*, xxxiii.

22. Cobb, *An Inquiry into the Law of Negro Slavery*, vol. 1, ccxii.

23. Smith, *Natural History of the Human Species*, 196.
24. Morton, *Crania Americana*, 88.
25. "Ethnology," *The Liberator*, July 9, 1858.
26. Walter, "Surviving in the Garret."
27. Jacobs, *Incidents in the Life of a Slave Girl*, 22.
28. Carby, *Reconstructing Womanhood*, 54. See also Sorisio, *Fleshing Out America*, 215.
29. Child, *The History of the Condition of Women*, 265.
30. Bourne, *Slavery Illustrated*, 87.
31. Jacobs, *Incidents in the Life of a Slave Girl*, 22.
32. Jacobs, *Incidents in the Life of a Slave Girl*, 218. Emphasis is original.
33. Jacobs, *Incidents in the Life of a Slave Girl*, 217.
34. Jacobs, *Incidents in the Life of a Slave Girl*, 217–18.
35. Jacobs, *Incidents in the Life of a Slave Girl*, 59.
36. Child, *The Mother's Book*, 153.
37. Child, *The Mother's Book*, 153.
38. Jacobs, *Incidents in the Life of a Slave Girl*, 44, 51.
39. Jacobs, *Incidents in the Life of a Slave Girl*, 53–54.
40. Jacobs, *Incidents in the Life of a Slave Girl*, 53–54.
41. Jacobs, *Incidents in the Life of a Slave Girl*, 53–54.
42. Tyler, *Disabilities of the Color Line*, 3–4.
43. Smith, *Self-Discovery and Authority*.
44. Carby, *Reconstructing Womanhood*, 47; Cogan, *All-American Girl*.
45. Herndl, "Invisible (Invalid) Woman." See also Foster, "Harriet Jacobs's *Incidents* and the 'Careless Daughters.'"
46. See Herndl, "Invisible (Invalid) Woman"; Fishburn, *The Problem of Embodiment in Early African American Narrative*; Kreiger, "Playing Dead"; Gomaa, "Writing to 'Virtuous' and 'Gentle' Readers."
47. Child, *The Mother's Book*, 143.
48. Jacobs, *Incidents in the Life of a Slave Girl*, 173.
49. Jacobs, *Incidents in the Life of a Slave Girl*, 174.
50. Jacobs, *Incidents in the Life of a Slave Girl*, 183.
51. Jacobs, *Incidents in the Life of a Slave Girl*, 224.
52. Titus, "'This Poisonous System,'" 205.
53. J.D., "Strange and Not Strange," *North Star*, February 23, 1849. "J.D." may refer to the African American abolitionist James W. Duffin, who lived in New York while Douglass was publishing the *North Star*.
54. "Exercise," *North Star*, May 4, 1849.
55. "Fresh Air," *Frederick Douglass' Paper*, March 4, 1852.
56. Child, *The Family Nurse*, 6, 40.
57. "Selections," *National Anti-Slavery Standard*, March 17, 1853.
58. Jacobs, *Incidents in the Life of a Slave Girl*, 174.
59. Jacobs, *Incidents in the Life of a Slave Girl*, 174, 175, 179.
60. Morgan, *Laboring Women*.
61. Hartman, *Scenes of Subjection*.
62. Fishburn, *The Problem of Embodiment in Early African American Narrative*.

63. Boster, *African American Slavery and Disability*.
64. Jacobs, *Incidents in the Life of a Slave Girl*, 199.
65. Jacobs, *Incidents in the Life of a Slave Girl*, 200.
66. Jacobs, *Incidents in the Life of a Slave Girl*, 200.
67. Jacobs, *Incidents in the Life of a Slave Girl*, 39.
68. Jacobs, *Incidents in the Life of a Slave Girl*, 228.
69. Jacobs, *Incidents in the Life of a Slave Girl*, 228.
70. Jacobs, *Incidents in the Life of a Slave Girl*, 235.
71. Jacobs, *Incidents in the Life of a Slave Girl*, 242.
72. Joshua Coffin to Lydia Maria Child, June 25, 1842, in Yellin, ed., *The Harriet Jacobs Family Papers*, vol. 1, 42.
73. Jacobs, *Incidents in the Life of a Slave Girl*, 254.
74. Child, *An Appeal in Favor of That Class of Americans Called Africans*, 85.
75. Fett, *Working Cures*, 18.
76. Walters, "Crip Mammy."
77. Jacobs, *Incidents in the Life of a Slave Girl*, 254–55.
78. Cope, "'I Verily Believed Myself to Be a Free Woman,'" 6.
79. On Jacobs's economic negotiations, see Diran, "Scenes of Speculation." On disability and labor in the nineteenth century, see Rose, *No Right to Be Idle*.
80. Jacobs, *Incidents in the Life of a Slave Girl*, 262.
81. Jacobs, *Incidents in the Life of a Slave Girl*, 290.
82. Jacobs, *Incidents in the Life of a Slave Girl*, 5.
83. Willis, *Out-Doors at Idlewild*, 464.
84. Willis, *Out-Doors at Idlewild*, 275–76.
85. Willis, *Out-Doors at Idlewild*, 292; Jacobs, *Incidents in the Life of a Slave Girl*, 185.
86. Harriet Jacobs to Amy Post, March 1854, in *Jacobs Family Papers*, vol. 1, 282; Harriet Jacobs to Amy Post, July 31, 1854, in *Jacobs Family Papers*, vol. 1, 221; Harriet Jacobs to Amy Post, May 18 and June 8, 1857, in *Jacobs Family Papers*, vol. 1, 235.
87. Harriet Jacobs to Amy Post, in *Jacobs Family Papers*, vol. 1, 221; Harriet Jacobs to Amy Post, December 27, 1854, in *Jacobs Family Papers*, vol. 1, 223.
88. Harriet Jacobs to Amy Post, August 7, 1855, in *Jacobs Family Papers*, vol. 1, 226.
89. Harriet Jacobs to Amy Post, March 1854, in *Jacobs Family Papers*, vol. 1, 213.
90. Jacobs, *Incidents in the Life of a Slave Girl*, 48.
91. Jacobs, *Incidents in the Life of a Slave Girl*, 303.
92. Harriet Jacobs to Amy Post, June 21, 1857, in *Jacobs Family Papers*, vol. 1, 237.
93. Manning, *Troubled Refuge*.
94. Downs, *Sick from Freedom*, 22.
95. Child, *The Freedmen's Book*, 218.
96. Downs, *Sick from Freedom*, 6.
97. Harriet Jacobs, quoted in "Report of Friends' Association," March 22, 1864, in *Jacobs Family Papers*, vol. 2, 556.
98. Harriet Jacobs, "Life among the Contrabands," in *Jacobs Family Papers*, vol. 2, 400.
99. Jacobs, "Life among the Contrabands," vol. 2, 404.
100. Downs, *Sick from Freedom*, 40.
101. Child, *The Freedmen's Book*, 246.

102. Long, *Doctoring Freedom*.

103. Jacobs, "Life among the Contrabands," vol. 2, 400.

104. See Harriet Jacobs, May 27, 1863, quoted in "The Second Report of a Committee of the Representatives of New York Yearly Meeting of Friends upon the Condition and Wants of the Colored Refugees," in *Jacobs Family Papers*, vol. 2, 486; and Jacobs, quoted in "Report of Friends' Association," vol. 2, 556.

105. Harriet Jacobs, quoted in "Fourth Report of a Committee of Representatives of New York Yearly Meeting of Friends upon the Condition and Wants of the Colored Refugees," May 1865, in *Jacobs Family Papers*, vol. 2, 629.

106. Lydia Maria Child, "Colored Refugees in Our Camps," in *Jacobs Family Papers*, vol. 2, 468.

107. Child, *The Family Nurse*, 6. Emphasis is mine.

108. Child, "Colored Refugees in Our Camps," in *Jacobs Family Papers*, vol. 2, 468.

109. "Jacobs School," February 1865, in *Jacobs Family Papers*, vol. 2, 613.

110. "Jacobs School," vol. 2, 613.

111. Donkor, "Laboring Bodies," 59.

112. Jacobs, "Life among the Contrabands," vol. 2, 400.

113. Spillers, "Mama's Baby, Papa's Maybe," 72. For further work on race science and sexual differentiation, see Wiegman, *American Anatomies*; Schuller, *The Biopolitics of Feeling*.

114. Spillers, "Mama's Baby, Papa's Maybe," 62.

115. Erevelles, *Disability and Difference in Global Contexts*, 41.

116. Jacobs, "Life among the Contrabands," vol. 2, 400.

117. Jacobs, "Life among the Contrabands," vol. 2, 401.

118. Harriet Jacobs to Lydia Maria Child, March 18, 1863, quoted in Child, "Colored Refugees in Our Camps," vol. 2, 470. See also Harriet Jacobs to H. Sella Martin, April 14, 1863, in *Jacobs Family Papers*, vol. 2, 477. Sewing also facilitated Jacobs's involvement in the abolitionist movement: in 1848 she joined the Rochester Ladies' Anti-Slavery Society's sewing circle to fundraise for the cause. See Hewitt, *Women's Activism and Social Change*.

119. Jacobs, "Life among the Contrabands," vol. 2, 404–5.

120. Keckley, *Behind the Scenes*, 113.

121. Hatton, "Biographical Sketch," 7.

122. Jacobs, "Life among the Contrabands," vol. 2, 405–6, emphasis mine.

123. Jacobs, *Incidents in the Life of a Slave Girl*, 127.

124. Jacobs, *Incidents in the Life of a Slave Girl*, 156. Jacobs's brother, John S. Jacobs, who went on to become a prominent abolitionist, offers a similar account in "A True Tale of Slavery" (1861), published in the London periodical *The Leisure Hour*. While, echoing *Incidents*, he recalls of his sister, "when she was sick, I visited her, and gave her such medicines as she needed," he reveals that such doctoring was not uncommon for him. Because he had previously been owned by Dr. James Norcom (Dr. Flint in *Incidents*), John's master (and the father of his sister's children) determined that he was "quite capable of visiting the sick slaves on the plantation." John S. Jacobs, "A True Tale of Slavery," in *Jacobs Family Papers*, vol. 1, 308.

125. Jacobs, *Incidents in the Life of a Slave Girl*, 145.

126. Mitchell, *From Slave Cabins to the White House*, 2, 3.
127. Jacobs, quoted in Child, "Colored Refugees in Our Camps," vol. 2, 469.
128. Jacobs, quoted in Child, "Colored Refugees in Our Camps," vol. 2, 469.
129. Mitchell, *From Slave Cabins to the White House*, 2.
130. Mitchell, *From Slave Cabins to the White House*, 38.
131. Jacobs, "Life among the Contrabands," vol. 2, 404–5.
132. Jacobs, quoted in "Fourth Report," vol. 2, 629.
133. Harriet Jacobs to Hannah Stevenson, March 10, 1864, in *Jacobs Family Papers*, vol. 2, 553. Hannah Stevenson was a white abolitionist who volunteered in Union hospitals.
134. Baumgartner, *In Pursuit of Knowledge*, 90.
135. After her mother's death in 1897, Louisa became a "matron" herself, first at the National Home for the Relief of Destitute Colored Women and Children and then at Howard University, where she had earlier taught in the industrial department.
136. H. Carter, "Extracts of Letters from Teachers," *The Freedmen's Record*, January 1, 1865.
137. Yellin, *Harriet Jacobs*, 208. Frances Harper briefly describes a similar school in her Reconstruction-Era novel, *Minnie's Sacrifice* (1869), when the character Louis announces, "We are going to open a school, and devote our lives to the upbuilding of the future race. . . . I believe there is power and capacity, only let it have room for exercise and development." Harper, *Minnie's Sacrifice, Sowing and Reaping, Trial and Triumph*, 73.
138. Harper, *Iola Leroy*, 147.
139. Harper, *Iola Leroy*, 199.
140. Louisa Jacobs to Ednah Dow Cheney, March 26, 1866, in *Jacobs Family Papers*, vol. 2, 667.
141. In *Incidents*, too, Jacobs describes "Ellen" (Louisa's pseudonym) as "sick" under slavery at the plantation and physically "neglected" by the cousins of the Willis family who first house her in the North.
142. Jacobs to Stevenson, March 10, 1864, in *Jacobs Family Papers*, vol. 2, 553.
143. Harriet Jacobs, letter, January 13, 1865, in *Jacobs Family Papers*, vol. 2, 611.
144. "Teachers," *The Freedmen's Record*, September 1, 1865. In 1866, the *Record* further clarified the utility of health to a teacher. Again listing the "1st [sic]" qualification for the position as "Health," the authors explain that it is needed "to a degree which will ensure energy, cheerfulness, and courage. These may come from the spirit, but at the cost of life itself, unless a sound body makes them natural and easy." "The Situation," *The Freedmen's Record*, July 1, 1866.
145. Harper, *Iola Leroy*, 200.
146. Harriet Jacobs, April 9, 1864, quoted in "Third Report of a Committee of Representatives of New York Yearly Meeting of Friends upon the Condition and Wants of the Colored Refugees," May 1864, in *Jacobs Family Papers*, vol. 2, 566.
147. Jacobs to Post, August 7, 1855, vol. 1, 226.
148. Knadler, *Vitality Politics*, 18; Carmody, "In Spite of Handicaps." On Black women's health activism in the post-Reconstruction era, see Smith, *Sick and Tired of Being Sick and Tired*.
149. Snorton, *Black on Both Sides*, 58.

Chapter Four

1. "Why Indian Children Die So Young," *The Indian Helper*, May 8, 1896.

2. Adams, *Education for Extinction*, 133; Woolford, *This Benevolent Experiment*, 235–38.

3. Throughout this chapter, I refer to "settler" rather than "white" educators in order to avoid the conflation of colonial and racialized powers that Jodi Byrd (Chickasaw Nation of Oklahoma) explains obfuscates Native assertions of sovereignty. Byrd, *The Transit of Empire*, xxiv.

4. Schuller, *The Biopolitics of Feeling*. As Ann Laura Stoler has famously shown, imperial education is a crucial site for understanding biopower's disciplinary influence, since it promoted a "set of behaviors that prescribed restraint and civility" and defined bourgeois adulthood in racialized terms. Stoler, *Race and the Education of Desire*, 151. On biopower and settler colonialism in the Americas, see Rifkin, "Indigenizing Agamben"; Morgensen, "The Biopolitics of Settler Colonialism."

5. Enoch, *Refiguring Rhetorical Education*, 86.

6. Lomawaima, "Domesticity in the Federal Indian Schools," 230, 232. As Susan Bernardin argues, Zitkala-Ša reveals the violence of this pedagogy by depicting the domestication of supposedly "savage" "squaws" as threats to Indigenous ways of life. Bernardin, "The Lessons of a Sentimental Education."

7. Morgensen, "The Biopolitics of Settler Colonialism," 56.

8. Ben-Moshe, *Decarcerating Disability*.

9. Cowing, "Occupied Land Is an Access Issue," 11. For an account of the continued wielding of rehabilitative logic against Indigenous youth in contemporary North America, see Chapman, "Colonialism, Disability, and Possible Lives."

10. Pratt, *Battlefield and Classroom*, 303.

11. Recognizing physical education as a pervasive feature of assimilationist education provides a crucial complement to the history of athletic programs for Native boys, especially Carlisle's famous football team. John Bloom, who has written extensively about boarding school sports, acknowledges the limitations of an overemphasis on this legacy, writing that "the inspiring stories of triumph and success associated with the Carlisle football and track teams can easily mask the fundamental pain and destruction created by assimilation policies." Bloom, "The Imperial Gridiron," 125.

12. My use of debility is drawn from Jasbir Puar, who differentiates this term from both "disability" and "impairment." "Debility," she explains, refers to "injury and bodily exclusion that are endemic rather than epidemic or exceptional." Puar, *The Right to Maim*, xvii.

13. Standing Bear, *My People the Sioux*, 164.

14. Cowing, "Occupied Land Is an Access Issue," 11.

15. For additional critiques of the social model of disability, see especially Shildrick and Price, *Vital Signs*; Siebers, *Disability Theory*; Erevelles, *Disability and Difference in Global Contexts*; Kafer, *Feminist, Queer, Crip*.

16. Schalk and Kim, "Integrating Race, Transforming Feminist Disability Studies," 42.

17. I refer to the author as "Zitkala-Ša" ("Red Bird") throughout this chapter because this is how she identifies herself in the publications I examine here. On the use of other names during Zitkala-Ša's life, including Gertrude Simmons and

Gertrude Bonnin (her married name), see Dominguez, "The Gertrude Bonnin Story," 8–12. In addition, I follow Mandy Suhr-Sytsma in identifying Zitkala-Ša as a "Yankton" writer. While, as Suhr-Sytsma notes, Zitkala-Ša's characters refer to themselves as "Indian" or, referencing their larger linguistic group membership, "Dakota," her lifelong ties to the specific Yankton Nation in South Dakota where she was born feature prominently in her writing and provide crucial context for her portrayals of Indigenous communities. Suhr-Sytsma, "Spirits from Another Realm."

18. Following Lucy Maddox, my reading of Zitkala-Ša's writings in the early 1900s is dually situated. Because she published these pieces immediately upon her departure from Carlisle, which concluded her decades-long immersion in educational institutions, my reading is situated primarily alongside the pedagogical theories and politics of off-reservation boarding schools. At the same time, however, I recognize the significance of Zitkala-Ša's decision to republish the pieces alongside newer works in the 1921 collection *American Indian Stories*. As Maddox points out, these newer additions were "specifically *about* reform work and specifically addressed to an audience of reform-minded (white) women," suggesting that Zitkala-Ša "saw the early work as relevant to the efforts of organizations like the [Society for American Indians] and the Women's Clubs to secure rights for American Indians, especially the rights of citizenship." Like Maddox, I read Zitkala-Ša's writing as engaged with the intersecting agendas of early twentieth-century Indigenous and women's reform movements. Maddox, *Citizen Indians*, 142. On the ethnographic quality of her 1900 stories, see Rifkin, *Speaking for the People*.

19. Kelsey, "Disability and Native North American Boarding School Narratives," 200.

20. Cowing, "Crip Interventions in Zitkála-Šá's Boarding School Stories," 219.

21. "Before" photographs showed students in tribal garb, while "after" images depicted them in the European-style military uniforms they were required to wear at the school. Photographs also often documented the cutting of students' hair, a practice Zitkala-Ša details in "School Days of an Indian Girl." For more on photography at Carlisle, see Wexler, *Tender Violence*; Mauro, *The Art of Americanization at the Carlisle Indian School*.

22. Burch, *Committed*, 10.

23. Teuton, "Disability in Indigenous North America," 574. See also Woolford, *This Benevolent Experiment*, 241.

24. Hailmann, *Report of the Indian School Superintendent*, 7.

25. "Eighteenth Annual Report of the Indian Industrial School at Carlisle, Penna."

26. Thompson introduced football, a sport the school would become known for, to Carlisle in 1894, and he served as head coach briefly before becoming disciplinarian. Thompson left his post in 1907, frustrated that the overemphasis on football had turned Carlisle into "a school of professional athletics" and that, as a result, "the discipline at the school ha[d] degenerated." "W. G. Thompson, 74, Educator, Is Dead," *New York Times*, March 31, 1940. W. G. Thompson to Carlos Montezuma, quoted in Jenkins, *The Real All Americans*, 243.

27. He later traveled with some of the youngest prisoners to Hampton Institute in Virginia, where they were enrolled alongside the school's African American pupils.

28. Pratt, *Battlefield and Classroom*, 155.

29. Mauro, *The Art of Americanization at the Carlisle Indian School*, 4–5. See also Bederman, *Manliness and Civilization*.

30. Roosevelt, "Christian Citizenship," 322, 331.

31. Roosevelt, "Christian Citizenship," 332.

32. "Why Indians Die," *The Indian Helper*, December 2, 1898.

33. "Why Indians Die."

34. "Why Indians Die."

35. "Why Indians Die."

36. Quoted in Enoch, *Refiguring Rhetorical Education*, 97.

37. Katanski, *Learning to Write Indian*, 51. For more on student writing at Carlisle, see also Enoch, *Refiguring Rhetorical Education*; Zink, "Carlisle's Writing Circle"; Klotz, *Writing Their Bodies*.

38. Katanski, *Learning to Write Indian*, 65.

39. "A Fourteen Year Old Girl's Good Advice," *The Indian Helper*, November 12, 1886.

40. Lomawaima, "Estelle Reel," 13. Much of the instruction published in Reel's *Course* also appeared in her first annual report. See United States Superintendent of Indian Schools, *Report of the Superintendent of Indian Schools*; Hailmann, *Report of the Indian School Superintendent*.

41. Schuller, *The Trouble with White Women*, 83; Henderson, *Settler Feminism and Race Making in Canada*; Arvin, "Indigenous Feminist Notes."

42. Trennert, "Educating Indian Girls at Nonreservation Boarding Schools."

43. Reel, *A Course of Study*, 148. On the kind of "nuclear family homemaking" such as Carlisle students were trained in as an invalidation of "alternative modes of inhabitance and landedness" as well as sovereignty, see Rifkin, *Settler Common Sense*, 28. On domesticity as a colonial apparatus in the West, see Simonsen, *Making Home Work*.

44. Reel, *A Course of Study*, 148.

45. Zaborskis, *Queer Childhoods*, 197.

46. Reel, *A Course of Study*, 148.

47. Pratt, *Battlefield and Classroom*, 312, 214.

48. Reel, *A Course of Study*, 190.

49. Jackson, "The Value of the Outing System for Girls," 864.

50. Reel, *A Course of Study*, 190.

51. Josephine E. Richards, "The Training of the Indian Girl as the Uplifter of the Home," *National Education Association Journal of Proceedings and Addresses* 39 (1900): 702.

52. Richards, "The Training of the Indian Girl," 701.

53. Richards, "The Training of the Indian Girl," 704.

54. Reel, *A Course of Study*, 197.

55. Reel, quoted in Lomawaima, "Domesticity in the Federal Indian Schools," 234.

56. "The Exercise That Makes Healthy Girls," *The Indian Helper*, February 2, 1900. This entry was reprinted from the *Ohio Chronicle*.

57. *The Indian Helper*, February 4, 1898.

58. Beecher, *A Treatise on Domestic Economy* rev., 131.

59. *Minutes of Indiana Yearly Meeting of Friends*, 1891, 20.

60. Nathan Coggeshall, quoted in Spack, "Dis/Engagement," 184.

61. Zitkala-Ša, "School Days," in *American Indian Stories, Legends, and Other Writings*, 89.
62. Zitkala-Ša, "School Days," 93.
63. Zitkala-Ša, "School Days," 90.
64. Zitkala-Ša, "School Days," 90.
65. Redmond, "The Sartorial Indian." For more on Zitkala-Ša's rhetorical manipulation of her own physical presentation when speaking publicly on behalf of Indigenous rights, see Spack, "Re-Visioning Sioux Women."
66. Zitkala-Ša, "Impressions," in *American Indian Stories, Legends, and Other Writings*, 69.
67. Zitkala-Ša, "Impressions," 86.
68. Zitkala-Ša, "School Days," 90.
69. Zitkala-Ša, "School Days," 90.
70. Zitkala-Ša, "School Days," 90.
71. Zitkala-Ša, "School Days," 93.
72. Zitkala-Ša, "School Days," 93.
73. Zitkala-Ša, "School Days," 93.
74. Zitkala-Ša, "School Days," 93.
75. Zitkala-Ša, "School Days," 95–96.
76. Zitkala-Ša, "School Days," 96.
77. Zitkala-Ša, "School Days," 96.
78. Zitkala-Ša, "School Days," 96.
79. Zitkala-Ša, "School Days," 96.
80. Burt, "'Death beneath This Semblance of Civilization,'" 79.
81. Zitkala-Ša, "School Days," 86.
82. Zitkala-Ša, "School Days," 86.
83. Zitkala-Ša, "School Days," 96.
84. Zitkala-Ša, "School Days," 96–97. As Tiffany Aldrich MacBain argues, Zitkala-Ša figures the settler body itself through its "metonymic connection to contagion and death." MacBain, "Cont(r)acting Whiteness," 57.
85. Zitkala-Ša, "An Indian Teacher," in *American Indian Stories, Legends, and Other Writings*, 112.
86. Cowing, "Crip Interventions in Zitkála-Šá's Boarding School Stories," 226.
87. Zitkala-Ša, "An Indian Teacher," in *American Indian Stories, Legends, and Other Writings*, 104, 105. Positioning herself first as an "Indian Girl" and later as an "Indian Teacher" heightens Zitkala-Ša's critique of boarding schools' rehabilitative aims by undermining the ideal trajectory of a "civilized" girl who spreads the domestic scientific knowledge she has acquired throughout her community. Lewandowski, *Red Bird, Red Power*, 27.
88. Zitkala-Ša, "An Indian Teacher," 106.
89. Zitkala-Ša, "An Indian Teacher," 106.
90. Zitkala-Ša, "An Indian Teacher," 112.
91. Quoted in *Sixty-Second Annual Report*, 452; Bloom, *To Show What an Indian Can Do*, 10. For more on displays of assimilationist education, see Trennert, "Selling Indian Education at World's Fairs and Expositions."

92. Zitkala-Ša, "An Indian Teacher," 104.

93. Zitkala-Ša, "An Indian Teacher," 105–6.

94. Zitkala-Ša, "A Protest against the Abolition of the Indian Dance," in *American Indian Stories, Legends, and Other Writings*, 237.

95. Zitkala-Ša, "A Protest against the Abolition of the Indian Dance," 237.

96. Zitkala-Ša, "A Protest against the Abolition of the Indian Dance," 237.

97. For more on the Canton Asylum see Burch, *Committed*.

98. Zitkala-Ša, "A Protest against the Abolition of the Indian Dance," 237.

99. Ben-Moshe, *Decarcerating Disability*, 1.

100. Zitkala-Ša further elaborates on such Indigenous parental training in the story "A Warrior's Daughter," published in *Everybody's Magazine* in 1902. The story opens with the protagonist, Tusee, "taking her first dancing lesson," and Zitkala-Ša depicts her comportment as a carefully choreographed and studied form. Zitkala-Ša echoes Reel's claim in *A Course of Study* that music "unites the physical, mental, and spiritual." However, the instruction depicted in "A Warrior's Daughter" is a distinctly Indigenous form of physical education that counters educators' claims that Native students' homes were injurious environments. Zitkala-Ša, "A Warrior's Daughter," in *American Indian Stories, Legends, and Other Writings*, 132.

101. Zitkala-Ša, "An Indian Teacher," 112.

102. Zitkala-Ša, "An Indian Teacher," 109.

103. Zitkala-Ša, "Impressions," 69.

104. Zitkala-Ša, "Why I Am a Pagan," *Atlantic Monthly*, December 1902, 801. Alex Henkle argues that river imagery here and in Zitkála-Šá's 1900 *Atlantic* stories reflects "the intricate dynamics of memory" and the ways in which colonialism has disrupted her connection to Dakota oral traditions in which rivers figure prominently. Henkle, "Leaves on the Trees," 134.

105. Zitkala-Ša, "Why I Am a Pagan," 802.

106. Zitkala-Ša, "Why I Am a Pagan," 802.

107. Cowing, "Crip Interventions in Zitkála-Šá's Boarding School Stories," 227.

108. Senier, "Disability, Blackness, and Indigeneity," 168.

109. Teuton, "Disability in Indigenous North America," 571.

110. Zitkala-Ša, "Impressions," 68.

111. Teuton, "Disability in Indigenous North America," 584.

112. Teuton, "Disability in Indigenous North America," 576.

113. Zitkala-Ša, "Why I Am a Pagan," 803; Zitkala-Ša, "School Days," 95.

114. Zitkala-Ša, "Why I Am a Pagan," 803.

115. Zitkala-Ša, "Why I Am a Pagan," 803.

116. Pratt, quoted in Katanski, *Learning to Write Indian*, 128.

117. Zitkala-Ša to Carlos Montezuma, April 13, 1901, in Lewandowski, *Red Bird, Red Power*, 52.

118. Zitkala-Ša to Montezuma, April 13, 1901, in Lewandowski, *Red Bird, Red Power*, 52.

119. Kelsey, "Disability and Native North American Boarding School Narratives," 197.

120. Pratt, *Battlefield and Classroom*, 303; Zitkala-Ša, "School Days," 96.

Chapter Five

1. Bancroft, *School Gymnastics, Free Hand*, 18.
2. Bancroft, *School Gymnastics, Free Hand*, 19.
3. Bancroft, *School Gymnastics, Free Hand*, 20.
4. Verbrugge, *Active Bodies*.
5. Remley, "Bancroft, Jessie Hubbell," 46–47.
6. Grimm, "Forerunners for a Domestic Revolution."
7. Deegan, "Introduction," 19.
8. Addams, "Recreation as a Public Function in Urban Communities," in *The Jane Addams Reader*, 616.
9. Davis, *Charlotte Perkins Gilman*, 183.
10. Davis, *Charlotte Perkins Gilman*, 184.
11. Smith-Rosenberg, *Disorderly Conduct*, 236.
12. McCrary, "From Hull-House to Herland."
13. Addams, "Woman and the State," 10.
14. Charlotte Perkins Gilman, "The Work Before Us," *The Forerunner*, January 1912, 8. As Deborah M. de Simone argues, Gilman "wrote about education and she wrote to educate" the general public. Simone, "Charlotte Perkins Gilman and Educational Reform," 146.
15. Weinbaum, "Writing Feminist Genealogy"; Seitler, *Atavistic Tendencies*; Lamp and Cleigh, "A Heritage of Ableist Rhetoric in American Feminism from the Eugenics Period"; Nadkarni, *Eugenic Feminism*; Tavera, "Her Body, Herland."
16. Charlotte Perkins Gilman, "Comment and Review," *The Forerunner*, December 1910, 25.
17. Addams, *Twenty Years at Hull-House*, 186.
18. Addams, *Twenty Years at Hull-House*, 231–32.
19. Ladd-Taylor, *Mother-Work*, 4–5.
20. Charlotte Perkins Gilman, "Our Overworked Instincts," *The Forerunner*, December 1910.
21. Gibson and Jung, "Historical Census Statistics on the Foreign-Born Population of the United States."
22. Up until the 1917 Immigration Act barred their entry, many came from Asia as well, though Chinese immigration was restricted beginning with the Chinese Exclusion Act of 1882.
23. Dolmage, *Disabled upon Arrival*, 25; Baynton, *Defectives in the Land*, 2.
24. Quoted in Dolmage, *Disabled upon Arrival*, 15.
25. Quoted in Dolmage, *Disabled upon Arrival*, 14.
26. Quoted in Ordover, *American Eugenics*, 7.
27. Quoted in Dolmage, *Disabled upon Arrival*, 35.
28. Quoted in Dolmage, *Disabled upon Arrival*, 17.
29. Quoted in Baynton, *Defectives in the Land*, 15.
30. Quoted in Ordover, *American Eugenics*, 8.
31. Prescott F. Hall, "Immigration Restriction and World Eugenics," *Journal of Heredity* 10, no. 3 (1919): 126.

32. Quoted in Baker, "The Racist Anti-Racism of American Anthropology," 132.

33. Sussman, *The Myth of Race*, 158.

34. *Pittsburgh Post*, quoted in Baker, "The Racist Anti-Racism of American Anthropology," 135.

35. Baker, "The Racist Anti-Racism of American Anthropology," 135.

36. Though radical in his rejection of racial determinism for European immigrants, Boas did not apply this same logic to non-white racial groups. He announced in W. E. B. Du Bois's *The Crisis* in 1912, "I do not believe that the negro is in his physical and mental make-up, the same as the European," and in the same speech he insisted "there is . . . no proof whatever that these differences signify any appreciable degree of inferiority of the negro, notwithstanding the slightly inferior size, and perhaps lesser complexity of structure, of his brain" (quoted in Baker, "The Racist Anti-Racism of American Anthropology," 137).

37. Boas, *Changes in Bodily Form of Descendants of Immigrants*, 26.

38. Boas, *Changes in Bodily Form of Descendants of Immigrants*, 26.

39. Hall, "Immigration Restriction and World Eugenics," 126.

40. Verbrugge, *Active Bodies*, 60.

41. Boas, *Changes in Bodily Form of Descendants of Immigrants*, 2.

42. Crampton, *The Pedagogy of Physical Training*, xi.

43. Crampton, *The Pedagogy of Physical Training*, xii, xiii.

44. Crampton, *The Pedagogy of Physical Training*, xiii.

45. Crampton, *The Pedagogy of Physical Training*, xiii.

46. Sargent, *Dudley Allen Sargent*, xiv.

47. Sargent, *Physical Education*, 22.

48. Sargent, *Physical Education*, 23.

49. Sargent, *Physical Education*, 126; Dudley Allen Sargent, "The Significance of a Sound Physique," *Annals of the American Academy of Political and Social Science* 34, no. 1 (1909): 14.

50. Dudley Allen Sargent, "The Place for Physical Training in the School and College Curriculum," *American Physical Education Review* 5, no. 1 (1900): 6, 17.

51. Sargent, *Dudley Allen Sargent*, 197.

52. Sargent, *Physical Education*, 247.

53. Charlotte Perkins Gilman, "The Providence Ladies Gymnasium," *Provincial Daily Journal*, May 23, 1883.

54. Charlotte Perkins Gilman, "Comment and Review," *The Forerunner*, January 1911. Though she criticized Sargent's use of "masculine" to describe what she considered "human" traits, she also repeatedly cited his anthropometric studies "made from gymnasium measurements of thousands of young collegians" as evidence of the disabilities imposed on women.

55. Harriet Park Thomas to Jane Addams, December 16, 1916, Jane Addams Digital Edition, https://digital.janeaddams.ramapo.edu/.

56. Hines, "'They Do Not Know How to Play,'" 211.

57. Knight, *Jane Addams*, 66. Addams and Starr modeled their settlement after London's Toynbee Hall, though that institution was led by men and focused primarily on men's clubs. The success of Addams and Starr's endeavor ignited the settlement

movement in the United States, which grew from six institutions in 1891 to over a hundred in 1900 and, by 1910, over four hundred. Jackson, *Lines of Activity*, 4.

58. Schneiderhan, "Pragmatism and Empirical Sociology," 612.
59. Addams, *Twenty Years at Hull-House*, 168–69.
60. Addams, "The Objective Value of a Social Settlement," 40.
61. Addams, "The Objective Value of a Social Settlement," 40.
62. Jackson, *Lines of Activity*, 73. The Mary Crane Nursery was run by the Chicago Relief and Aid Society in conjunction with Hull-House. The project was the "result of a conference held at Hull-House in regard to the lack of adequate day nursery accommodations in Chicago." "Hull-House Year Book 1906–1907," 44.
63. Jane Addams to Rose Marie Gyles, July 8, 1904, Jane Addams Digital Edition.
64. Quoted in Hines, "'They Do Not Know How to Play,'" 218.
65. *Bulletin*. In 1914, the Chicago School for Playground Workers became the Recreation Department of the Chicago School of Civics and Philanthropy (of which Addams was a board member) from 1914 to 1920. For more on Boyd, see Boyd and Simon, *Play and Game Theory in Group Work*.
66. On Dewey's and Addams's shared investments in pragmatism beyond the progressive education movement, see Seigfried, "Socializing Democracy."
67. Addams, "Home and the Special Child," in *The Jane Addams Reader*, 226.
68. Addams, "Home and the Special Child," 226.
69. Addams, "Home and the Special Child," 224.
70. Jane Addams, "The Children of the Nation," *Ladies' Home Journal*, September 1912.
71. Jackson, *Lines of Activity*, 116.
72. Addams, *Democracy and Social Ethics*, 185.
73. Addams, "Americanization," 246.
74. Addams, "Americanization," 246.
75. Addams, *Twenty Years at Hull-House*, 103.
76. Cooper, *The Autobiography of Citizenship*, 122.
77. Addams, *Twenty Years at Hull-House*, 443–44.
78. Addams, *Twenty Years at Hull-House*, 91.
79. Jane Addams, "Recreation as a Public Function in Urban Communities," *American Journal of Sociology* 17, no. 5 (1912): 617.
80. Addams, "Recreation as a Public Function," in *The Jane Addams Reader*, 616–17.
81. Addams, "Recreation as a Public Function," 619.
82. Addams, "Recreation as a Public Function," 619.
83. Addams, *Twenty Years at Hull-House*, 231–32.
84. Ladd-Taylor, *Mother-Work*, 79.
85. Addams, "Recreation as a Public Function," 619.
86. "Let Children Play, Says Jane Addams," *St. Louis Star and Times*, March 25, 1911, 7.
87. Jane Addams, "The Juvenile Adult Offender," *Ladies' Home Journal* 30 (October 1913): 24.
88. Addams, "The Juvenile Adult Offender," 24.
89. Jane Addams, "Miss Addams," *Ladies' Home Journal* 30 (May 1913): 27.
90. Addams, "Miss Addams," 27.

91. Addams, "Miss Addams," 27.
92. Addams, "Miss Addams," 27.
93. Addams, quoted in "Let Children Play, Says Jane Addams," 7.
94. Jane Addams, "Miss Addams," *Ladies' Home Journal* 30 (July 1913): 19. For an account of working-class young women's recreation that emphasizes the experiences and perspective of participants themselves, see Peiss, *Cheap Amusements*; McBee, *Dance Hall Days*.
95. Addams, *A New Conscience and an Ancient Evil*, 110.
96. Addams, *The Spirit of Youth and the City Streets*, 20.
97. Addams, *The Spirit of Youth and the City Streets*, 6. This statement also appeared in the year before *The Spirit of Youth* was published, in a 1908 column in *Playground* magazine. Jane Addams, "Miss Addams Said," *Playground* (April 1908): 26.
98. Addams, *The Spirit of Youth and the City Streets*, 92.
99. Addams, *The Spirit of Youth and the City Streets*, 95.
100. Addams, *Twenty Years at Hull-House*, 442.
101. Addams, *Twenty Years at Hull-House*, 442.
102. Salazar, *Bodies of Reform*, 235.
103. Addams, *Twenty Years at Hull-House*, 442.
104. Addams, quoted in "Let Children Play, Says Jane Addams," 7.
105. Hines, *Lines of Activity*, 217.
106. Addams, "Public School and the Immigrant Child," in *The Jane Addams Reader*, 236.
107. Addams, "Public School and the Immigrant Child," 236.
108. Jane Addams, "Some Reflections on the Failure of the Modern City to Provide Recreation for Young Girls," *Charities and the Commons* 21 (December 5, 1908): 368. A slightly altered version of this same anecdote also appeared one year later in Addams, *The Spirit of Youth and the City Streets*, 102.
109. Addams, "Some Reflections on the Failure of the Modern City," 368.
110. Addams, "Some Reflections on the Failure of the Modern City," 368.
111. Addams, *Twenty Years at Hull-House*, 442.
112. Addams, *A New Conscience and an Ancient Evil*, 131.
113. Addams, *A New Conscience and an Ancient Evil*, 131.
114. On working young women's actual sexual expression, see Peiss, *Cheap Amusements*, 108–12.
115. Quoted in Davis, *Charlotte Perkins Gilman*, 178.
116. Deegan, "Introduction," 19.
117. Deegan, "Introduction," 23; Hill, *Charlotte Perkins Gilman*, 275. In 1897, when Gilman spent an extended period in Chicago, she lived with Marietta Dow, whose daughter, Gilman's close friend Jennie Dow, was Hull-House's first kindergarten teacher.
118. Gilman, *The Living of Charlotte Perkins Gilman*, 186.
119. Abate, *Tomboys*; Salazar, *Bodies of Reform*.
120. Gilman, *Moving the Mountain*.
121. Charlotte Perkins Gilman, "Prize Children," *The Forerunner*, May 1910.
122. Gilman, "Prize Children."
123. Gilman, *Women and Economics*, vii.

124. In *Concerning Children* (1903), Gilman speculates that although biologist August Weissman claimed "mutilations" were not heritable, positive traits produced by "a long, slow, cautious, delicate but inexorable system of exercise" could be transmissible. She describes a hypothetical experiment on the effects of healthy habits on guinea pigs, which she invoked again in her novel *What Diantha Did*, published in *The Forerunner* from 1909 to 1910. Gilman, *Concerning Children*, 12–13.

125. Charlotte Perkins Gilman, "A Small God and a Large Goddess," *The Forerunner*, November 1909, 2.

126. Gilman, *The Living of Charlotte Perkins Gilman*, 28.

127. Studley, *What Our Girls Ought to Know*, 250–51.

128. Blaikie, *How to Get Strong and How to Stay So*, 113.

129. Gilman, *Women and Economics*, 194. Gilman herself had a complicated relationship with motherhood and eventually sent her own daughter, Katharine, to be raised by her ex-husband, Walter Stetson, and his second wife. As her biographer Cynthia J. Davis puts it, "for Gilman, mothering and career never mixed well or smoothly." Davis, "Concerning Children," 110.

130. Simone, "Charlotte Perkins Gilman and Educational Reform," 135.

131. Gilman, *Women and Economics*, 193, 195.

132. On the relationship between Gilman's and Beecher's ideas about motherhood, see Elbert, "The Sins of the Mothers."

133. Gilman, *Women and Economics*, 197.

134. Gilman, *The Home, Its Work and Influence*, 334–35.

135. Gilman, "A Garden of Babies," 130.

136. Gilman "A Garden of Babies," 134.

137. Gilman "A Garden of Babies," 135.

138. Gilman, *The Crux*, 271. The instructor's nationality is noteworthy here, as it suggests a familiarity with the "Swedish method" of gymnastics, which was highly popular when Gilman was writing in the 1910s.

139. Gilman, *The Crux*, 271.

140. Gilman, *The Crux*, 32.

141. Gilman, *The Crux*, 276.

142. Charlotte Perkins Gilman, "The New Motherhood," *The Forerunner*, December 1910, 17; Gilman, *Concerning Children*, 269.

143. Charlotte Perkins Gilman, "Teaching the Mothers," *The Forerunner*, March 1912, 74.

144. Gilman, *Concerning Children*, 133.

145. Gilman, *Concerning Children*, 134.

146. Gilman, *Moving the Mountain*, 104.

147. Gilman, *Moving the Mountain*, 108, 106.

148. Gilman, *Moving the Mountain*, 104–5.

149. Gilman, *Moving the Mountain*, 108, 197.

150. Gilman, *Moving the Mountain*, 197.

151. Gilman, *Moving the Mountain*, 211.

152. Gilman, *Moving the Mountain*, 211, 212.

153. Gilman, *Moving the Mountain*, 211, 213.

154. While Herland's all-female population might appear to offer an opportunity to integrate queerness into ideas about physical culture, the notion of same-sex attraction is seemingly foreclosed by the novel's insistence that all the nation's citizens are "sisters." Indeed, while both Addams and Gilman engaged in romantic relationships with women, neither addresses queerness in their writings about women's attention to embodiment. This silence reflects the anxieties about lesbianism and female masculinity among those who trained future physical education teachers in turn-of-the-century normal schools. Worried about what the Department of Physical Education for Women at the University of Wisconsin–Madison called "the 'crush' situation" among pupils, educators across the country worked to instill a feminine code of "Phy Ed-iquette" in physical education students that they believed would facilitate their heterosexuality. Verbrugge, *Active Bodies*, 23–25.

155. Garland-Thomson, "Welcoming the Unbidden," 82.

156. Gilman, "Herland," 83.

157. Gilman, "Herland," 24, 34, 130. Indeed, as Abate suggests, it may be the remarkable bodily mastery that the Herlanders have already cultivated through physical activity that enables them to voluntarily control their parthenogenesis.

158. Gilman, "Herland," 34.

159. Gilman, "Herland," 83.

160. McCrary, "From Hull-House to Herland," 76; Gilman, "Herland," 84.

161. Gilman, "Herland," 96.

162. Gilman, "Herland," 107.

163. Gilman, "Herland," 104.

164. Gilman, "Herland," 107.

165. Gilman, "Herland," 108.

166. Gilman, "Herland," 108.

167. Gilman, "Herland," 108.

168. Gilman, "Herland," 108.

169. Gilman, "Herland," 108.

170. Gilman, "Herland," 108.

171. Gilman, "Herland," 65.

172. Gilman, "Herland," 34.

173. Gilman, "Herland," 132, 34.

174. Gilman, "Herland," 34.

175. Charlotte Perkins Gilman, "Is America Too Hospitable?," *Forum*, October 1923. See also Knight, "Charlotte Perkins Gilman and the Shadow of Racism," 159–69.

176. Gilman, "Is America Too Hospitable?"

177. Charlotte Perkins Gilman, "Immigration, Importation, and Our Fathers," *The Forerunner*, May 1914, 118.

178. Gilman, *Concerning Children*, 55. Susan Lanser makes note of this claim in her reading of *The Yellow Wall Paper* but does not connect it to Gilman's broader concerns about child-culture. Lanser, "Feminist Criticism," 429.

179. Gilman, *With Her in Ourland*, 93.

180. Gilman, *Concerning Children*, 12. For similar invocations of foot binding in Gilman's work, see also Gilman, *The Home, Its Work and Influence*, 154; Gilman,

The Man-Made World, 165; Gilman, *With Her in Ourland*, 93; and Gilman, *The Dress of Women*, 32.

181. Gilman, *With Her in Ourland*, 98, 97.
182. Gilman, *With Her in Ourland*, 97.
183. Nadkarni, *Eugenic Feminism*, 35.
184. Gilman, *With Her in Ourland*, 109.
185. Gilman, *With Her in Ourland*, 113.
186. Gilman, *With Her in Ourland*, 121.
187. Gilman, *With Her in Ourland*, 99.
188. Gilman, "Immigration, Importation, and Our Fathers," 118.
189. Gilman, "Immigration, Importation, and Our Fathers," 119.
190. Gilman, "Immigration, Importation, and Our Fathers," 119.
191. Gilman, *Moving the Mountain*, 52, 55.
192. See Gilman, *The Man-Made World*.
193. Bederman, *Manliness and Civilization*, 156.
194. Gilman, "Herland," 132.
195. Gilman, "Herland," 132.
196. Gilman, "Herland," 140. Emphasis is original.
197. Charlotte Perkins Gilman, "A Suggestion on the Negro Problem," *American Journal of Sociology* 14, no. 1 (1908): 80, 81.
198. Gilman, "A Suggestion on the Negro Problem," 79–80.
199. Gilman, "A Suggestion on the Negro Problem," 80, 81.
200. Gilman, "A Suggestion on the Negro Problem," 81.
201. Gilman, "A Suggestion on the Negro Problem," 83.
202. Gilman, "A Suggestion on the Negro Problem," 82, 80.
203. For historical perspectives on the relationship between disability and criminality through the lens of incarceration, see Ben-Moshe, Chapman, and Carey, eds., *Disability Incarcerated*. On the role of muscular development in Gilman's ideas about morality and character formation, see Salazar, *Bodies of Reform*.
204. Charlotte Perkins Gilman, "Mending Morals by Making Muscle," *Saturday Evening Post*, May 19, 1900.
205. Gilman, "Mending Morals by Making Muscle." Gilman shared this perspective with Sargent, who argued that "in the treatment of criminals, dullards and the mentally defective, who have as a class very poor physiques, it has been found necessary to reconstruct and improve them physically as far as possible by systematic exercise, bathing, dieting, etc., before they can be much improved mentally and morally." Sargent, "The Significance of a Sound Physique," 14.
206. Gilman, *Moving the Mountain*, 259.
207. Gilman, *Herland*, 112. Jennifer Hudak suggests that "sending the patient to bed" resembles the "rest cure" Gilman underwent under the supervision of Silas Weir Mitchell. Hudak, "The Social Inventor," 473–74. Given Gilman's critique of the rest cure in *The Yellow Wall Paper*, such an echo potentially unsettles her general presentation of Herland's government as an aspirational feminist ideal.
208. Gilman, "A Suggestion on the Negro Problem," 83.
209. Gilman, "A Suggestion on the Negro Problem," 83.

210. Hudak, "The Social Inventor," 472.
211. Gilman, "Immigration, Importation, and Our Fathers," 118.

Epilogue

1. Margaret Abrams, "You Can Now Buy a 'Wellness' Self-Care Barbie Which Comes with Gym Clothes and a Protein Bar," *Business Insider*, February 4, 2020, https://www.businessinsider.com/wellness-self-care-barbie-gym-wear-spa-products-pajamas-launch-2020-2.
2. Ashley Oerman, "Barbie Is Doing 'Self-Care' Now, and I Think We've Gone Too Far," *Cosmopolitan*, January 30, 2020, https://www.cosmopolitan.com/health-fitness/a30718416/wellness-barbie-mattel/.
3. Hannah Smothers, "New Wellness Barbies Lead Children to the Gruesome Altar of Self-Care," *Vice*, January 31, 2020, https://www.vice.com/en/article/g5xy4b/wellness-barbie-self-care.
4. On wellness influencers more broadly, see Lawrence, ed., *Digital Wellness, Health and Fitness Influencers*.
5. "Statistics & Facts," Global Wellness Institute, accessed January 24, 2023, https://globalwellnessinstitute.org/press-room/statistics-and-facts/.
6. Deena Shakir, quoted in Brooke DiPalma, "'The Dollars Are Massive' When You Invest in Women's Health, Venture Capitalist Says," *Yahoo! Finance*, March 19, 2022, https://finance.yahoo.com/news/womens-health-dollars-venture-capitalist-184909152.html.
7. Tolentino, "Always Be Optimizing"; Marisa Meltzer, "Why Wellness Is the New Way to Look, Feel, and Act Rich," *The Cut*, July 18, 2016, https://www.thecut.com/swellness/2016/07/why-wellness-is-the-new-luxury-lifestyle-status-symbol.html.
8. Taffy Brodesser-Akner, "How Goop's Haters Made Gwyneth Paltrow's Company Worth $250 Million," *New York Times Magazine*, July 25, 2018, https://www.nytimes.com/2018/07/25/magazine/big-business-gwyneth-paltrow-wellness.html.
9. Dunn, "What High-Level Wellness Means," 447. Emphasis is original.
10. Dunn, "What High-Level Wellness Means," 447. Emphasis is original.
11. Tolentino, "Always Be Optimizing," 81.
12. Laurie Penny, "Life-Hacks of the Poor and Aimless," *The Baffler*, July 8, 2016, https://thebaffler.com/war-of-nerves/laurie-penny-self-care. See also Tolentino, "Always Be Optimizing," 93–94.
13. Crawford, "Healthism and the Medicalization of Everyday Life," 368.
14. Jackie Chiquoine, "The Effects of COVID-19 on the Wellness Industry," US Chamber of Commerce, August 11, 2020, https://www.uschamber.com/co/co/good-company/launch-pad/pandemic-is-changing-wellness-industry.
15. Amanda Hess, "Our Health Is in Danger. Wellness Wants to Fill the Void," *New York Times*, April 6, 2020, https://www.nytimes.com/2020/04/06/arts/virus-wellness-self-care.html.
16. Baker, "Alt. Health Influencers."
17. Tan et al., "Association between Income Inequality and County-Level COVID-19 Cases and Deaths."

18. Amy Larocca, "In a Pandemic, Is 'Wellness' Just Being Well-Off?," *The Cut*, April 29, 2020, https://www.thecut.com/2020/04/wellness-during-coronavirus.html.

19. Kirkland, "Critical Perspectives on Wellness," 980.

20. Mickey, "'"Eat, Pray, Love" Bullshit,'" 105.

21. McIntyre et al., "The Dubious Empirical and Legal Foundations of Wellness Programs," 90; Till, "Creating 'Automatic Subjects,'" 418–35; J. Wortham, "The Rise of the Wellness App," *New York Times Magazine*, February 17, 2021, https://www.nytimes.com/2021/02/17/magazine/wellness-apps.html.

22. Tolentino, "Always Be Optimizing," 76; Caitlin Flanagan, "Sheryl Sandberg and the Crackling Hellfire of Corporate America," *The Atlantic*, June 18, 2022, https://www.theatlantic.com/ideas/archive/2022/06/sheryl-sandberg-leaving-meta-lean-in-feminism/661291/.

23. Rittu Sinha, "How and Why Women Can and Should Prioritize Their Wellness," *Forbes*, October 25, 2022, https://www.forbes.com/sites/forbescoachescouncil/2022/10/25/how-and-why-women-can-and-should-prioritize-their-wellness/.

24. Grigg and Kirkland, "Health," 341.

25. Amy Larocca, "How 'Wellness' Became an Epidemic," *The Cut*, June 27, 2017, https://www.thecut.com/2017/06/how-wellness-became-an-epidemic.html.

26. Brodesser-Akner, "How Goop's Haters Made Gwyneth Paltrow's Company Worth $250 Million."

27. Raphael, *The Gospel of Wellness*.

28. Maya Dusenbery has shown that a wide range of chronic conditions such as autoimmune diseases, fibromyalgia, chronic fatigue syndrome, chronic Lyme disease, and multiple chemical sensitivities are all most common in women, and all are relatively neglected in medical research and practice. Dusenbery, *Doing Harm*, 3. On how this systemic neglect drives women to the wellness industry, see Raphael, *The Gospel of Wellness*.

29. On the role of self-care in these feminist health organizations, see Kline, *Bodies of Knowledge*, 9–40; Schalk, *Black Disability Politics*, 82–92. On women's leadership roles in the Black Panther Party's health programs such as the Free Breakfast Program, see Nelson, *Body and Soul*, 88–90, 96; Bloom, *Black against Empire*, 181–85, 193–94. See also Aisha Harris, "A History of Self-Care," *Slate*, April 5, 2017, http://www.slate.com/articles/arts/culturebox/2017/04/the_history_of_self_care.html.

30. See, for example, Penny, "Life-Hacks of the Poor and Aimless"; Marisa Meltzer, "Soak, Steam, Spritz: It's All Self-Care," *New York Times*, December 10, 2016, https://www.nytimes.com/2016/12/10/fashion/post-election-anxiety-self-care.html; Jordan Kisner, "The Politics of Conspicuous Displays of Self-Care," *New Yorker*, March 14, 2017, https://www.newyorker.com/culture/culture-desk/the-politics-of-selfcare; Christianna Silva, "The Millennial Obsession with Self-Care," *NPR*, June 4, 2017, https://www.npr.org/2017/06/04/531051473/the-millennial-obsession-with-self-care; Hess, "Our Health Is in Danger." Notably, many of these pieces were published leading up to and in the wake of the 2016 presidential election, when many claimed that Donald Trump's victory prompted a spike in attention to self-care, especially among women.

31. Lorde, *A Burst of Light*, 130.

32. Kim and Schalk, "Reclaiming the Radical Politics of Self-Care," 327.

33. Lorde, *The Collected Poems of Audre Lorde*, 125.

34. O'Neill, "Pursuing 'Wellness,'" 632.

35. "Have You Tried Yoga?," accessed January 11, 2023, https://haveyoutriedyoga
podcast.wordpress.com/. Raphael, too, titled the first chapter of her book on wellness culture "Why the Hell Is the Advice Always Yoga?"

36. Huber, *Pain Woman Takes Your Keys*, 25.

37. Huber, *Pain Woman Takes Your Keys*, 26.

38. Huber, *Pain Woman Takes Your Keys*, 48, 26.

39. Huber, *Pain Woman Takes Your Keys*, 26–27.

40. Fariha Róisín, "At All Costs," *Harper's Bazaar*, May 17, 2022, https://www.harpersbazaar.com/culture/features/a39697817/at-all-costs-may-2022/.

41. Róisín, *Who Is Wellness For?*, 44.

42. Róisín, *Who Is Wellness For?*, 37.

43. Róisín, *Who Is Wellness For?*, 159.

44. Megan Falk, "What's the Deal with the Ayurvedic Diet?," *Shape*, June 4, 2020, https://www.shape.com/healthy-eating/diet-tips/ayurvedic-diet-guide.

45. Róisín, *Who Is Wellness For?*, 159.

46. "Studio Ānanda," accessed February 2, 2023, https://www.studioananda.space/.

47. "About—Jessamyn Stanley," accessed February 2, 2023, https://jessamynstanley.com/about/.

48. Stanley, *Yoke*, 13.

49. Stanley, *Yoke*, 17.

50. Stanley, *Every Body Yoga*, ix.

51. Stanley, *Yoke*, 163.

52. Stanley, *Yoke*, 163. On how the slender ideal of white femininity was developed in concert with anti-Blackness, see Strings, *Fearing the Black Body*.

53. Friedman, *Let's Get Physical*, 240. Emphasis is mine.

54. Stanley, *Yoke*, 165.

55. Stanley, *Yoke*, 165.

56. Hersey, *Rest Is Resistance*, 26.

57. In identifying her project as "womanist," Hersey draws on a long tradition of Black women's radical thought. Defining womanist in 1983, Alice Walker invokes well-being by imagining "a black feminist or feminist of color" who is "committed to survival and wholeness of entire people." Walker, *In Search of Our Mothers' Gardens*, xi.

58. Hersey, *Rest Is Resistance*, 4. Throughout *Rest Is Resistance* Hersey uses the term "DreamSpace" to refer to a mental state in which one can "envision a world centered in justice" (11).

59. Hersey, *Rest Is Resistance*, 5, 8.

60. Hersey, *Rest Is Resistance*, 83–84.

61. Hersey, *Rest Is Resistance*, 25.

62. Hersey, *Rest Is Resistance*, 16.

63. Hersey, *Rest Is Resistance*, 63.

64. Hersey, *Rest Is Resistance*, 12.

65. Hersey, *Rest Is Resistance*, 67.

66. Hersey, *Rest Is Resistance*, 24–25.

67. Hersey, *Rest Is Resistance*, 61, 17.

Bibliography

Primary Sources

Archive

Jane Addams Digital Edition

Periodicals

American Journal of Sociology
American Physical Education Review
Annals of the American Academy of Political and Social Science
Atlantic/Atlantic Monthly
Baffler
Business Insider
Charities and the Commons
Cosmopolitan
Cut
Forbes
Forerunner
Forum
Frederick Douglass' Paper
Freedmen's Record
Harper's Bazaar
Indian Helper
Journal of Heredity
Ladies' Home Journal
Monthly Repository
National Anti-Slavery Standard
National Education Association Journal of Proceedings and Addresses
New Yorker
New York Times
North Star
Playground
Provincial Daily Journal
Saturday Evening Post
Shape
Slate
St. Louis Star and Times
Vice
Yahoo! Finance

Books

Addams, Jane. "Americanization." In *The Jane Addams Reader*, edited by Jean Bethke Elshtain, 240–47. New York: Basic Books, 2008.
———. *Democracy and Social Ethics*. New York: Macmillan, 1902.
———. *A New Conscience and an Ancient Evil*. New York: Macmillan, 1912.
———. "The Objective Value of a Social Settlement." In *The Jane Addams Reader*, edited by Jean Bethke Elshtain, 29–45. New York: Basic Books, 2008.
———. *The Spirit of Youth and the City Streets*. New York: Macmillan, 1909.
———. *Twenty Years at Hull-House with Autobiographical Notes*. New York: Macmillan, 1910.
———. "Woman and the State." Speech before the New York Women's Political Union, February 12, 1911.
Alcott, Amos Bronson. *Observations on the Principles and Methods of Infant Instruction*. Boston: Carter & Hendee, 1830.

Alcott, Louisa May. *Little Men: Life at Plumfield with Jo's Boys*. Boston: Roberts Brothers, 1871.

Bancroft, Jessie Hubbell. *School Gymnastics, Free Hand: A System of Physical Exercises for Schools*. New York: E. L. Kellogg, 1896.

Beaujeu, J. A. *A Treatise on Gymnastic Exercises: Or, Calisthenics for the Use of Young Ladies: Introduced at the Royal Hibernian Military School, Also at the Seminary for the Education of Young Ladies, under the Direction of Miss Hincks in 1824*. Dublin: R. Milliken, 1828.

Beecher, Catharine Esther. *Letters to Persons Who Are Engaged in Domestic Service*. New York: Leavitt & Trow, 1842.

———. *Suggestions Respecting Improvements in Education: Presented to the Trustees of the Hartford Female Seminary, and Published at Their Request*. Hartford, CT: Packard & Butler, 1829.

———. *A Treatise on Domestic Economy: For the Use of Young Ladies at Home, and at School*. Boston: Marsh, Capen, Lyon, and Webb, 1841.

———. *A Treatise on Domestic Economy: For the Use of Young Ladies at Home, and at School*, rev. ed. New York: Harper & Brothers, 1843.

Beecher, Catharine Esther, and Harriet Beecher Stowe. *The American Woman's Home, or, Principles of Domestic Science: Being a Guide to the Formation and Maintenance of Economical, Healthful, Beautiful, and Christian Homes*. New York: J. B. Ford, 1869.

Blaikie, William. *How to Get Strong and How to Stay So*. New York: Harper & Brothers, 1879.

Boas, Franz. *Changes in Bodily Form of Descendants of Immigrants*. Washington, DC: US Government Printing Office, 1911.

Bourne, George. *Slavery Illustrated in Its Effects upon Woman and Domestic Society*. Boston: Isaac Knapp, 1837.

Boyd, Neva Leona. *Play and Game Theory in Group Work; a Collection of Papers*. Chicago: Jane Addams Graduate School of Social Work, University of Illinois at Chicago Circle, 1971.

"Bulletin." Chicago School of Civics and Philanthropy, 1914.

Child, Lydia Maria. *An Appeal in Favor of That Class of Americans Called Africans*. Boston: Allen and Ticknor, 1833.

———. *The Family Nurse: Or, Companion of the Frugal Housewife*. Boston: C. J. Hendee, 1837.

———. *The Freedmen's Book*. Boston: Ticknor and Fields, 1865.

———. *The History of the Condition of Women, in Various Ages and Nations*. Boston: J. Allen, 1835.

———. *The Mother's Book*. Boston: Carter, Hendee, and Babcock, 1831.

Cobb, Thomas R. R. *An Inquiry into the Law of Negro Slavery in the United States of America*, vol. 1. Philadelphia: T. & J. W. Johnson, 1858.

Cooper, James Fenimore. *Correspondence of James Fenimore-Cooper*. 2 vols. New Haven, CT: Yale University Press, 1922.

A Course of Calisthenics for Young Ladies, in Schools and Families. With Some Remarks on Physical Education. Hartford, CT: H. and F. J. Huntington, 1831.

Crampton, Charles Ward. *The Pedagogy of Physical Training, with Special Reference to Formal Exercises*. New York: Macmillan, 1922.

"Eighteenth Annual Report of the Indian Industrial School at Carlisle, Penna." Carlisle: Carlisle Indian School, 1897.

Emerson, Ralph Waldo. "The American Scholar." In *Emerson's Prose and Poetry*, edited by Saundra Morris and Joel Porte. New York: W. W. Norton, 2001.

———. "Nature." In *Emerson's Prose and Poetry*, edited by Saundra Morris and Joel Porte, 27–55. New York: W. W. Norton, 2001.

Emerson, Ralph Waldo, W. H. Channing, and James Freeman Clarke, eds. *Memoirs of Margaret Fuller Ossoli*. 3 vols. Boston: Phillips, Sampson, 1852.

Farrar, Eliza Ware. *The Young Lady's Friend*. Boston: American Stationers' Company, 1838.

Fuller, Margaret. "Autobiographical Romance." In *The Essential Margaret Fuller*, edited by Jeffrey Steele, 24–43. New Brunswick, NJ: Rutgers University Press, 1992.

———. *The Letters of Margaret Fuller: 1845–1847*. Edited by Robert N. Hudspeth. Ithaca, NY: Cornell University Press, 1987.

———. "Physical Education and the Preservation of Health." In *Margaret Fuller's New York Journalism: A Biographical Essay and Key Writings*, edited by Catherine C. Mitchell, 190–93. Knoxville: University of Tennessee Press, 1995.

———. *Summer on the Lakes, in 1843*. Boston: Charles C. Little, 1844.

———. *Woman in the Nineteenth Century*. New York: Greeley & McElrath, 1845.

———. "The Wrongs of American Women, The Duty of American Women." In *Margaret Fuller's New York Journalism: A Biographical Essay and Key Writings*, edited by Catherine C. Mitchell, 128–34. Knoxville: University of Tennessee Press, 1995.

Gilman, Charlotte Perkins. *Concerning Children*. Boston: Small, Maynard, 1903.

———. *The Crux: A Novel*. New York: Charlton, 1911.

———. *The Dress of Women: A Critical Introduction to the Symbolism and Sociology of Clothing*. Edited by Michael R. Hill and Mary Jo Deegan. Westport, CT: Greenwood Press, 2002.

———. "A Garden of Babies." In *Charlotte Perkins Gilman: Her Progress toward Utopia with Selected Writings*, by Carol Farley Kessler. Syracuse, NY: Syracuse University Press, 1995.

———. "Herland." In *The Yellow Wall-Paper, Herland, and Selected Writings*, edited by Denise D. Knight, 1–146. New York: Penguin Classics, 2009.

———. *The Home, Its Work and Influence*. New York: McClure, Phillips, 1903.

———. *The Living of Charlotte Perkins Gilman: An Autobiography*. Madison: University of Wisconsin Press, 1991.

———. *The Man-Made World: Or, Our Androcentric Culture*. New York: Charlton, 1914.

———. *Moving the Mountain*. New York: Charlton, 1911.

———. *What Diantha Did*. Edited by Charlotte J. Rich. Durham, NC: Duke University Press, 2005.

———. *With Her in Ourland: Sequel to Herland*. Edited by Mary Jo Deegan and Michael R. Hill. Westport, CT: Greenwood Press, 1997.

———. *Women and Economics: A Study of the Economic Relation between Men and Women as a Factor in Social Evolution*. Boston: Small, Maynard, 1898.

———. "The Work Before Us." *The Forerunner*, January 1912.

———. *The Yellow Wall Paper*. Boston: Small, Maynard, 1891.

Hailmann, W. H. *Report of the Indian School Superintendent to the Secretary of the Interior*. Washington, DC: US Government Printing Office, 1896.

Hall, Francis. *Travels in Canada, and the United States, in 1816 and 1817*. London: Longman, Hurst, Rees, Orme, and Brown, 1818.

Hall, Prescott F. "Immigration Restriction and World Eugenics." Boston: Immigration Restriction League, 1919.

Hamilton, Elizabeth. *Letters on Education*. London: G. G. and J. Robinson, 1801.

Harper, Frances Ellen Watkins. *Iola Leroy, Or, Shadows Uplifted*. Philadelphia: Garrigues, 1892.

———. *Minnie's Sacrifice, Sowing and Reaping, Trial and Triumph: Three Rediscovered Novels*. Edited by Frances Smith Foster. Boston: Beacon Press, 2000.

Hersey, Tricia. *Rest Is Resistance: A Manifesto*. New York: Little, Brown Spark, 2022.

Higginson, Thomas Wentworth. *Margaret Fuller Ossoli*. Boston: Houghton Mifflin, 1890.

Huber, Sonya. *Pain Woman Takes Your Keys, and Other Essays from a Nervous System*. Lincoln: University of Nebraska Press, 2017.

"Hull-House Year Book 1906–1907." Chicago: Hull-House, 1907.

Jackson, Laura. "The Value of the Outing System for Girls." *National Education Association Journal of Proceedings and Addresses* 41 (1902): 44–45.

Jacobs, Harriet A. *Incidents in the Life of a Slave Girl. Written by Herself*. Edited by Lydia Maria Child. Boston: Author, 1861.

Keckley, Elizabeth. *Behind the Scenes, Or, Thirty Years a Slave and Four Years in the White House*. New York: G. W. Carleton, 1868.

Locke, John. *Some Thoughts Concerning Education*. London: A. and J. Churchill, 1693.

Logan, John. *Sermons, by the Late Rev. John Logan, F.R.S.E. One of the Ministers of Leith. Including a Complete Detail of the Service of a Communion Sabbath, According to the Usage of the Church of Scotland. With a Life of the Author*. Edinburgh: Thomas Nelson, 1839.

Lorde, Audre. *A Burst of Light: And Other Essays*. Mineola, NY: Courier Dover, 2017.

———. *The Collected Poems of Audre Lorde*. New York: W. W. Norton, 2000.

Malthus, Thomas Robert. *An Essay on the Principle of Population, as It Affects the Future Improvements of Society*. London: J. Johnson, 1798.

Manning, Chandra. *Troubled Refuge: Struggling for Freedom in the Civil War*. New York: Vintage, 2017.

Martineau, Harriet. *Harriet Martineau's Autobiography*. 3 vols. London: Smith, Elder, 1877.

———. *How to Observe: Morals and Manners*. London: Charles Knight, 1838.

———. *Society in America*. 2 vols. New York: Saunders and Otley, 1837.

Minutes of Indiana Yearly Meeting of Friends. Richmond, IN: T. E. De Yarnd General Job Printer, 1891.

Moore, Margaret King, and Stephen Salisbury. *Advice to Young Mothers on the Physical Education of Children*. Boston: Hilliard, Gray, 1833.

Morton, Samuel George. *Crania Americana: Or a Comparative View of the Skulls of Various Aboriginal Nations of North and South America to Which Is Prefixed an Essay on the Varieties of the Human Species*. Philadelphia: J. Dobson, 1839.

Nichols, Mary Sargeant Gove. *Lectures to Women on Anatomy and Physiology: With an Appendix on Water Cure*. New York: Harper & Brothers, 1846.

Nott, Josiah Clark, and George R. Gliddon. *Types of Mankind: Or, Ethnological Researches, Based upon the Ancient Monuments, Paintings, Sculptures, and Crania of Races, and upon Their Natural, Geographical, Philological, and Biblical History*. Philadelphia: Lippincott, 1854.

Owen, Robert Dale, and Frances Wright. *Tracts on Republican Government and National Education: Addressed to the Inhabitants of the United States of America*. London: J. Watson, 1840.

Phelps, Almira Hart Lincoln. *Lectures to Young Ladies: Comprising Outlines and Applications of the Different Branches of Female Education, for the Use of Female Schools, and Private Libraries*. Boston: Carter, Hendee, 1833.

Plain Talk and Friendly Advice to Domestics: With Counsel on Home Matters. Boston: Phillips, Sampson, 1855.

Pratt, Richard Henry. *Battlefield and Classroom: Four Decades with the American Indian, 1867–1904*. Edited by Robert M. Utley. New Haven, CT: Yale University Press, 1964.

Proceedings of the Woman's Rights Convention, Held at West Chester, Pa., June 2d and 3d, 1852. Philadelphia: Merrihew and Thompson, 1852.

Reel, Estelle. *Course of Study for the Indian Schools of the United States. Industrial and Literary*. Washington, DC: US Government Printing Office, 1901.

Róisín, Fariha. *Who Is Wellness For? An Examination of Wellness Culture and Who It Leaves Behind*. New York: HarperCollins, 2022.

Roosevelt, Theodore. "Christian Citizenship." In *The Strenuous Life: Essays and Addresses*, 321–32. New York: Century, 1902.

Rousseau, Jean-Jacques. *Emile, or On Education*. Translated by Allan Bloom. New York: Basic Books, 1979.

Rush, Benjamin. *A Plan for the Establishment of Public Schools and the Diffusion of Knowledge in Pennsylvania; to Which Are Added Thoughts upon the Mode of Education, Proper in a Republic: Addressed to the Legislature and Citizens of the State*. Philadelphia: Thomas Dobson, 1786.

Sargent, Dudley Allen. *Dudley Allen Sargent: An Autobiography*. Edited by Ledyard W. Sargent. Philadelphia: Lea & Febiger, 1927.

———. *Physical Education*. Boston: Ginn & Company, 1906.

———. "The Significance of a Sound Physique." *Annals of the American Academy of Political and Social Science* 34, no. 1 (1909): 9–15.

Sedgwick, Catharine Maria. *Life and Letters of Catharine M. Sedgwick*. Edited by Mary E. Dewey. New York: Harper & Brothers, 1871.

———. *Live and Let Live: Or, Domestic Service Illustrated*. New York: Harper, 1837.

———. *Means and Ends: Or, Self-Training*, 2nd ed. New York: Harper & Brothers, 1842.

Sigourney, Lydia Howard. *Letters to Young Ladies*, 2nd ed. Hartford, CT: William Watson, 1835.

Sixty-Second Annual Report of the Commissioner of Indian Affairs to the Secretary of the Interior. Washington, DC: US Government Printing Office, 1893.

Smith, Charles Hamilton. *Natural History of the Human Species: Its Typical Forms, Primaeval Distribution Filiations and Migration*. Edinburgh: W. H. Lizars, 1848.

Society for the Encouragement of Faithful Domestic Servants of New York. *First Annual Report of the Society for the Encouragement of Faithful Domestic Servants in New-York*. New York: American Tract Society, 1826.

Standing Bear, Luther. *My People the Sioux*. Lincoln: University of Nebraska Press, 2006.

Stanley, Jessamyn. *Every Body Yoga: Let Go of Fear, Get On the Mat, Love Your Body*. New York: Workman, 2017.

———. *Yoke: My Yoga of Self-Acceptance*. New York: Workman, 2021.

Steinem, Gloria. *Moving beyond Words: Age, Rage, Sex, Power, Money, Muscles: Breaking Boundaries of Gender*. New York: Simon and Schuster, 1995.

Studley, Mary J. *What Our Girls Ought to Know*. New York: M. L. Holbrook, 1878.

Thoreau, Henry David. "Walden." In *Walden, Civil Disobedience, and Other Writings: Authoritative Texts, Journal, Reviews and Posthumous Assessments, Criticism*, edited by William John Rossi, 3rd ed. New York: W. W. Norton, 2008.

———. "Walking." In *Walden, Civil Disobedience, and Other Writings: Authoritative Texts, Journal, Reviews and Posthumous Assessments, Criticism*, edited by William John Rossi, 3rd ed. New York: W. W. Norton, 2008.

United States Superintendent of Indian Schools. *Report of the Superintendent of Indian Schools*. Washington, DC: US Government Printing Office, 1898.

Willard, Emma. *A Plan for Improving Female Education*, 2nd ed. Middlebury, VT: S. W. Copeland, 1819.

Willis, Nathaniel Parker. *Out-Doors at Idlewild*. New York: Charles Scribner, 1855.

Wilson, Harriet E. *Our Nig; or, Sketches from the Life of a Free Black in a Two-Story White House, North*. Boston: G. C. Rand & Avery, 1859.

Wollstonecraft, Mary. *A Vindication of the Rights of Woman: With Strictures on Political and Moral Subjects*. Dublin: J. Stockdale, 1793.

Wright, Frances. *A Lecture on Existing Evils and Their Remedy: As Delivered in the Arch Street Theatre, to the Citizens of Philadelphia, June 2, 1829*. New York: George H. Evans, 1829.

———. *Views of Society and Manners in America: In a Series of Letters from That Country to a Friend in England, during the Years 1818, 1819, and 1820*. London: Longman, Hurst, Rees, Orme, and Brown, 1821.

Zitkala-Ša. *American Indian Stories, Legends, and Other Writings*. Edited by Cathy N. Davidson and Ada Norris. New York: Penguin Classics, 2003.

Secondary Sources

Books

Abate, Michelle Ann. *Tomboys: A Literary and Cultural History*. Philadelphia: Temple University Press, 2008.

Adams, David Wallace. *Education for Extinction: American Indians and the Boarding School Experience, 1875–1928*, 3rd ed. Lawrence: University of Kansas Press, 1995.

Alaimo, Stacy. *Undomesticated Ground: Recasting Nature as Feminist Space*. Ithaca, NY: Cornell University Press, 2000.

Altschuler, Sari. *The Medical Imagination: Literature and Health in the Early United States*. Philadelphia: University of Pennsylvania Press, 2018.

Barclay, Jenifer L. *The Mark of Slavery: Disability, Race, and Gender in Antebellum America*. Urbana: University of Illinois Press, 2021.

Bartlett, Elizabeth Ann. *Liberty, Equality, Sorority: The Origins and Interpretation of American Feminist Thought: Frances Wright, Sarah Grimke, and Margaret Fuller*. Brooklyn, NY: Carlson, 1994.

Baumgartner, Kabria. *In Pursuit of Knowledge: Black Women and Educational Activism in Antebellum America*. New York: New York University Press, 2019.

Baym, Nina. *Novels, Readers, and Reviewers: Responses to Fiction in Antebellum America*. Ithaca, NY: Cornell University Press, 2018.

———. *Woman's Fiction: A Guide to Novels by and about Women in America, 1820–70*, 2nd ed. Urbana: University of Illinois Press, 1993.

Baynton, Douglas C. *Defectives in the Land: Disability and Immigration in the Age of Eugenics*. Chicago: University of Chicago Press, 2016.

Bederman, Gail. *Manliness and Civilization: A Cultural History of Gender and Race in the United States, 1880–1917*. Chicago: University of Chicago Press, 1995.

Ben-Moshe, Liat. *Decarcerating Disability: Deinstitutionalization and Prison Abolition*. Minneapolis: University of Minnesota Press, 2020.

Ben-Moshe, Liat, Chris Chapman, and Allison C. Carey, eds. *Disability Incarcerated: Imprisonment and Disability in the United States and Canada*. New York: Palgrave Macmillan, 2014.

Bernstein, Robin. *Racial Innocence: Performing American Childhood from Slavery to Civil Rights*. New York: New York University Press, 2011.

Bloom, John. "The Imperial Gridiron: Dealing with the Legacy of Carlisle Indian School Sports." In *Carlisle Indian Industrial School*, edited by Jacqueline Fear-Segal and Susan D. Rose, 124–38. Lincoln: University of Nebraska Press, 2016.

———. *To Show What an Indian Can Do: Sports at Native American Boarding Schools*. Minneapolis: University of Minnesota Press, 2000.

Bloom, Joshua. *Black against Empire: The History and Politics of the Black Panther Party*. Berkeley: University of California Press, 2016.

Boster, Dea H. *African American Slavery and Disability: Bodies, Property and Power in the Antebellum South, 1800–1860*. New York: Routledge, 2012.

Burbick, Joan. *Healing the Republic: The Language of Health and the Culture of Nationalism in Nineteenth-Century America*. New York: Cambridge University Press, 1994.

Burch, Susan. *Committed: Remembering Native Kinship in and beyond Institutions*. Chapel Hill: University of North Carolina Press, 2021.

Byrd, Jodi A. *The Transit of Empire: Indigenous Critiques of Colonialism*. Minneapolis: University of Minnesota Press, 2011.

Capper, Charles. *Margaret Fuller: An American Romantic Life*. 2 vols. New York: Oxford University Press, 1994.
Carby, Hazel V. *Reconstructing Womanhood: The Emergence of the Afro-American Woman Novelist*. New York: Oxford University Press, 1990.
Cogan, Frances. *All-American Girl: The Ideal of Real Womanhood in Mid-Nineteenth-Century America*. Athens: University of Georgia Press, 2010.
Cooper, Tova. *The Autobiography of Citizenship: Assimilation and Resistance in US Education*. New Brunswick, NJ: Rutgers University Press, 2015.
Cooper Owens, Deirdre. *Medical Bondage: Race, Gender, and the Origins of American Gynecology*. Athens: University of Georgia Press, 2018.
Davidson, Cathy N., and Jessamyn Hatcher, eds. *No More Separate Spheres! A Next Wave American Studies Reader*. Durham, NC: Duke University Press, 2002.
Davis, Cynthia. *Charlotte Perkins Gilman: A Biography*. Stanford, CA: Stanford University Press, 2010.
Deák, Gloria-Gilda. *Passage to America: Celebrated European Visitors in Search of the American Adventure*. London: I. B. Tauris, 2013.
Deegan, Mary Jo. "Introduction." In *With Her in Ourland: Sequel to Herland*, by Charlotte Perkins Gilman, edited by Michael R. Hill and Mary Jo Deegan. Westport, CT: Greenwood, 1997.
Dolmage, Jay. *Disabled upon Arrival: Eugenics, Immigration, and the Construction of Race and Disability*. Columbus: Ohio State University Press, 2018.
Dominguez, Susan Rose. "The Gertrude Bonnin Story: From Yankton Destiny into American History, 1804-1938." PhD dissertation, Michigan State University, 2005.
Donkor, Crystal S. "Laboring Bodies." In *The Cambridge Companion to the Black Body in American Literature*, edited by Cherene Sherrard-Johnson, 49-61. Cambridge: Cambridge University Press, 2024.
Doty, Josh. *The Perfecting of Nature: Reforming Bodies in Antebellum Literature*. Chapel Hill: University of North Carolina Press, 2020.
Downs, Jim. *Sick from Freedom: African-American Illness and Suffering during the Civil War and Reconstruction*. New York: Oxford University Press, 2012.
Duane, Anna Mae. *Suffering Childhood in Early America: Violence, Race, and the Making of the Child Victim*. Athens: University of Georgia Press, 2011.
Dudden, Faye E. *Serving Women: Household Service in Nineteenth-Century America*. Middletown, CT: Wesleyan University Press, 1985.
Dusenbery, Maya. *Doing Harm: The Truth about How Bad Medicine and Lazy Science Leave Women Dismissed, Misdiagnosed, and Sick*. New York: HarperOne, 2018.
Edelstein, Sari. *Adulthood and Other Fictions: American Literature and the Unmaking of Age*. Oxford: Oxford University Press, 2018.
Elbert, Monika. "The Sins of the Mothers and Charlotte Perkins Gilman's Covert Alliance with Catharine Beecher." In *Charlotte Perkins Gilman and Her Contemporaries: Literary and Intellectual Contexts*, edited by Cynthia J. Davis and Denise D. Knight, 103-26. Tuscaloosa: University Alabama Press, 2004.
Enoch, Jessica. *Refiguring Rhetorical Education: Women Teaching African American, Native American, and Chicano/a Students, 1865-1911*. Carbondale: Southern Illinois University Press, 2008.

Erevelles, Nirmala. *Disability and Difference in Global Contexts: Enabling a Transformative Body Politic*. New York: Palgrave Macmillan, 2011.
Fett, Sharla M. *Working Cures: Healing, Health, and Power on Southern Slave Plantations*. Chapel Hill: University of North Carolina Press, 2002.
Fielder, Brigitte. *Relative Races: Genealogies of Interracial Kinship in Nineteenth-Century America*. Durham, NC: Duke University Press, 2020.
Fish, Cheryl J. *Black and White Women's Travel Narratives: Antebellum Explorations*. Gainesville: University Press of Florida, 2004.
Fishburn, Katherine. *The Problem of Embodiment in Early African American Narrative*. Westport, CT: Greenwood Press, 1997.
Fisher, Laura R. *Reading for Reform: The Social Work of Literature in the Progressive Era*. Minneapolis: University of Minnesota Press, 2019.
Foreman, P. Gabrielle. *Activist Sentiments: Reading Black Women in the Nineteenth Century*. Urbana: University of Illinois Press, 2009.
———. "Introduction." In *Our Nig: Or, Sketches from the Life of a Free Black*, by Harriet E. Wilson, edited by Reginald Pitts. New York: Penguin, 2009.
Foster, Frances Smith. "Harriet Jacobs's Incidents and the 'Careless Daughters' (and Sons) Who Read It." In *The (Other) American Traditions: Nineteenth-Century Women Writers*, edited by Joyce W. Warren, 92–108. New Brunswick, NJ: Rutgers University Press, 1993.
Friedman, Danielle. *Let's Get Physical: How Women Discovered Exercise and Reshaped the World*. New York: Penguin, 2022.
Garland-Thomson, Rosemarie. *Extraordinary Bodies: Figuring Physical Disability in American Culture and Literature*. New York: Columbia University Press, 1997.
———. "Welcoming the Unbidden: A Case for Conserving Human Biodiversity." In *What Democracy Looks Like: A New Critical Realism for a Post-Seattle World*, edited by Amy Schrager Lang and Cecelia Tichi. New Brunswick, NJ: Rutgers University Press, 2006.
Gibson, Campbell, and Kay Jung. "Historical Census Statistics on the Foreign-Born Population of the United States: 1850 to 2000." Working paper, US Census Bureau, February 2006.
Gilmore, Susan. "Margaret Fuller 'Receiving' the Indians." In *Margaret Fuller's Cultural Critique: Her Age and Legacy*, edited by Fritz Fleischmann, 75–90. New York: Peter Lang, 2000.
Glenn, Evelyn Nakano. *Forced to Care: Coercion and Caregiving in America*. Cambridge, MA: Harvard University Press, 2010.
Goodlad, Lauren M. E. "Imperial Woman: Harriet Martineau, Geopolitics and the Romance of Improvement." In *Harriet Martineau: Authorship, Society and Empire*, edited by Ella Dzelzainis and Cora Kaplan, 197–213. Manchester: Manchester University Press, 2010.
Grigg, Amanda J., and Anna Kirkland. "Health." In *The Oxford Handbook of Feminist Theory*, edited by Lisa Disch and Mary Hawkesworth, 326–45. New York: Oxford University Press, 2018.
Harper, Lila Marz. *Solitary Travelers: Nineteenth-Century Women's Travel Narratives and the Scientific Vocation*. Madison, NJ: Fairleigh Dickinson University Press, 2001.

Hartman, Saidiya V. *Scenes of Subjection: Terror, Slavery, and Self-Making in Nineteenth-Century America*. Oxford: Oxford University Press, 1997.
Hatton, Louise. "Biographical Sketch." In *Maria W. Stewart, America's First Black Woman Political Writer: Essays and Speeches*, edited by Marilyn Richardson. Bloomington: Indiana University Press, 1987.
Hayden, Wendy. *Evolutionary Rhetoric: Sex, Science, and Free Love in Nineteenth-Century Feminism*. Carbondale: Southern Illinois University Press, 2013.
Haynes, April R. *Riotous Flesh: Women, Physiology, and the Solitary Vice in Nineteenth-Century America*. Chicago: University of Chicago Press, 2015.
Henderson, Jennifer Anne. *Settler Feminism and Race Making in Canada*. Toronto: University of Toronto Press, 2003.
Hewitt, Nancy A. *Women's Activism and Social Change: Rochester, New York, 1822–1872*. Ithaca, NY: Cornell University Press, 1984.
Hill, Mary Armfield. *Charlotte Perkins Gilman: The Making of a Radical Feminist, 1860–1896*. Philadelphia: Temple University Press, 1980.
Horowitz, Helen Lefkowitz. *Rereading Sex: Battles over Sexual Knowledge and Suppression in Nineteenth-Century America*. New York: Vintage Books, 2003.
Jackson, Holly. *American Radicals: How Nineteenth-Century Protest Shaped the Nation*. New York: Crown, 2019.
Jackson, Shannon. *Lines of Activity: Performance, Historiography, Hull-House Domesticity*. Ann Arbor: University of Michigan Press, 2000.
Jenkins, Sally. *The Real All Americans*. New York: Anchor, 2008.
Kafer, Alison. *Feminist, Queer, Crip*. Bloomington: Indiana University Press, 2013.
Katanski, Amelia V. *Learning to Write Indian*. Norman: University of Oklahoma Press, 2007.
Kissel, Susan S. *In Common Cause: The "Conservative" Frances Trollope and the "Radical" Frances Wright*. Bowling Green, OH: Bowling Green State University Popular Press, 1993.
Kline, Wendy. *Bodies of Knowledge: Sexuality, Reproduction, and Women's Health in the Second Wave*. Chicago: University of Chicago Press, 2010.
Klotz, Sarah. *Writing Their Bodies: Restoring Rhetorical Relations at the Carlisle Indian School*. Logan: Utah State University Press, 2021.
Knadler, Stephen. *Vitality Politics: Health, Debility, and the Limits of Black Emancipation*. Ann Arbor: University of Michigan Press, 2019.
Knight, Louise W. *Jane Addams: Spirit in Action*. New York: W. W. Norton, 2010.
Kolodny, Annette. *The Land before Her: Fantasy and Experience of the American Frontiers, 1630–1860*. Chapel Hill: University of North Carolina Press, 2014.
Ladd-Taylor, Molly. *Mother-Work: Women, Child Welfare, and the State, 1890–1930*. Urbana: University of Illinois Press, 1994.
Lamp, Sharon, and W. Carol Cleigh. "A Heritage of Ableist Rhetoric in American Feminism from the Eugenics Period." In *Feminist Disability Studies*, edited by Kim Q. Hall, 175–90. Bloomington: Indiana University Press, 2011.
Lawrence, Stefan, ed. *Digital Wellness, Health and Fitness Influencers: Critical Perspectives on Digital Guru Media*. New York: Routledge, 2022.

Levander, Caroline. *Cradle of Liberty: Race, the Child, and National Belonging from Thomas Jefferson to W. E. B. Du Bois*. Durham, NC: Duke University Press, 2006.

Lewandowski, Tadeusz. *Red Bird, Red Power: The Life and Legacy of Zitkala-Ša*. Norman: University of Oklahoma Press, 2016.

Logan, Dana W. *Awkward Rituals: Sensations of Governance in Protestant America*. Chicago: University of Chicago Press, 2022.

Long, Margaret Geneva. *Doctoring Freedom: The Politics of African American Medical Care in Slavery and Emancipation*. Chapel Hill: University of North Carolina Press, 2012.

Maddox, Lucy. *Citizen Indians: Native American Intellectuals, Race, and Reform*. Ithaca, NY: Cornell University Press, 2005.

Manion, Jen. *Liberty's Prisoners: Carceral Culture in Early America*. Philadelphia: University of Pennsylvania Press, 2015.

Manning, Chandra. *Troubled Refuge: Struggling for Freedom in the Civil War*. New York: Vintage, 2017.

Mauro, Hayes Peter. *The Art of Americanization at the Carlisle Indian School*. Albuquerque: University of New Mexico Press, 2011.

McBee, Randy. *Dance Hall Days: Intimacy and Leisure among Working-Class Immigrants in the United States*. New York: New York University Press, 2000.

Metzl, Jonathan M. "Why against Health?" In *Against Health: How Health Became the New Morality*, edited by Anna Kirkland and Jonathan M. Metzl, 1–11. New York: New York University Press, 2010.

Minich, Julie Avril. *Radical Health: Unwellness, Care, and Latinx Expressive Culture*. Durham, NC: Duke University Press, 2023.

Mitchell, Koritha. *From Slave Cabins to the White House: Homemade Citizenship in African American Culture*. Urbana: University of Illinois Press, 2020.

Morantz-Sanchez, Regina. *Sympathy and Science: Women Physicians in American Medicine*, 2nd ed. Chapel Hill: University of North Carolina Press, 1999.

More, Ellen S., Elizabeth Fee, and Manon Parry. *Women Physicians and the Cultures of Medicine*. Baltimore: Johns Hopkins University Press, 2009.

Morgan, Jennifer L. *Laboring Women: Reproduction and Gender in New World Slavery*. Philadelphia: University of Pennsylvania Press, 2011.

Nadkarni, Asha. *Eugenic Feminism: Reproductive Nationalism in the United States and India*. Minneapolis: University of Minnesota Press, 2014.

Nelson, Alondra. *Body and Soul: The Black Panther Party and the Fight against Medical Discrimination*. Minneapolis: University of Minnesota Press, 2011.

Oravec, Christine L. "Fanny Wright and the Enforcing of Prudence: Women, Propriety, and Transgression in the Nineteenth-Century Public Oratory of the United States." In *Prudence*, edited by Robert Hariman. University Park: Pennsylvania State University Press, 2003.

Ordover, Nancy. *American Eugenics: Race, Queer Anatomy, and the Science of Nationalism*. Minneapolis: University of Minnesota Press, 2003.

Peiss, Kathy Lee. *Cheap Amusements: Working Women and Leisure in Turn-of-the-Century New York*. Philadelphia: Temple University Press, 1986.

Phillips-Cunningham, Danielle T. *Putting Their Hands on Race: Irish Immigrant and Southern Black Domestic Workers*. New Brunswick, NJ: Rutgers University Press, 2019.

Puar, Jasbir K. *The Right to Maim: Debility, Capacity, Disability*. Durham, NC: Duke University Press, 2017.

Purkiss, Ava. *Fit Citizens: A History of Black Women's Exercise from Post-Reconstruction to Postwar America*. Chapel Hill: University of North Carolina Press, 2023.

Raphael, Rina. *The Gospel of Wellness: Gyms, Gurus, Goop, and the False Promise of Self-Care*. New York: Henry Holt, 2022.

Reiss, Benjamin. *Wild Nights: How Taming Sleep Created Our Restless World*. New York: Basic Books, 2017.

Remley, Mary L. "Bancroft, Jessie Hubbell." In *Notable American Women: The Modern Period: A Biographical Dictionary*, edited by Barbara Sicherman and Carol Hurd Green, 46–47. Cambridge, MA: Harvard University Press, 1980.

Rendell, Jane. "Prospects of the American Republic, 1795–1821: The Radical and Utopian Politics of Robina Millar and Frances Wright." In *Enlightenment and Emancipation*, edited by Susan Manning and Peter France, 145–59. Lewisburg, PA: Bucknell University Press, 2006.

Rifkin, Mark. *Settler Common Sense: Queerness and Everyday Colonialism in the American Renaissance*. Minneapolis: University of Minnesota Press, 2014.

———. *Speaking for the People: Native Writing and the Question of Political Form*. Durham, NC: Duke University Press, 2021.

Roberson, Susan L. "Geographies of Expansion: Nineteenth-Century Women's Travel Writing." In *Inventing Destiny: Cultural Explorations of US Expansion*, edited by Jimmy L. Bryan, 118–36. Lawrence: University Press of Kansas, 2019.

Roberts, Caroline. *The Woman and the Hour: Harriet Martineau and Victorian Ideologies*. Toronto: University of Toronto Press, 2002.

Roberts, Dorothy. *Killing the Black Body: Race, Reproduction, and the Meaning of Liberty*. New York: Vintage, 1998.

Romero, Lora. *Home Fronts: Domesticity and Its Critics in the Antebellum United States*. Durham, NC: Duke University Press, 1997.

Rose, Sarah F. *No Right to Be Idle: The Invention of Disability, 1840s–1930s*. Chapel Hill: University of North Carolina Press, 2017.

Rusert, Britt. *Fugitive Science: Empiricism and Freedom in Early African American Culture*. New York: New York University Press, 2017.

Ryan, Barbara. *Love, Wages, Slavery: The Literature of Servitude in the United States*. Urbana: University of Illinois Press, 2006.

Salazar, James B. *Bodies of Reform: The Rhetoric of Character in Gilded Age America*. New York: New York University Press, 2010.

Sánchez-Eppler, Karen. *Dependent States: The Child's Part in Nineteenth-Century American Culture*. Chicago: University of Chicago Press, 2005.

———. *Touching Liberty: Abolition, Feminism, and the Politics of the Body*. Berkeley: University of California Press, 1993.

Schalk, Sami. *Black Disability Politics*. Durham, NC: Duke University Press, 2022.

Schuller, Kyla. *The Biopolitics of Feeling: Race, Sex, and Science in the Nineteenth Century*. Durham, NC: Duke University Press, 2018.

———. *The Trouble with White Women: A Counterhistory of Feminism*. New York: Bold Type Books, 2021.
Schwartz, Marie Jenkins. *Birthing a Slave: Motherhood and Medicine in the Antebellum South*. Cambridge, MA: Harvard University Press, 2006.
Seitler, Dana. *Atavistic Tendencies: The Culture of Science in American Modernity*. Minneapolis: University of Minnesota Press, 2008.
Shapiro, Joe. *The Illiberal Imagination: Class and the Rise of the U.S. Novel*. Charlottesville: University of Virginia Press, 2017.
Shildrick, Margrit, and Janet Price. *Vital Signs: Feminist Reconfigurations of the Bio/Logical Body*. Edinburgh: Edinburgh University Press, 1998.
Siebers, Tobin. *Disability Theory*. Ann Arbor: University of Michigan Press, 2008.
Simone, Deborah M. de. "Charlotte Perkins Gilman and Educational Reform." In *Charlotte Perkins Gilman: Optimist Reformer*, edited by Jill Rudd and Val Gough, 128–47. Iowa City: University of Iowa Press, 1999.
Simonsen, Jane E. *Making Home Work: Domesticity and Native American Assimilation in the American West, 1860–1919*. Chapel Hill: University of North Carolina Press, 2006.
Singley, Carol J. "Servitude and Homelessness: Harriet Wilson's Our Nig." In *Adopting America: Childhood, Kinship, and National Identity in Literature*, edited by Carol J. Singley. Oxford University Press, 2011.
Smith, Susan Lynn. *Sick and Tired of Being Sick and Tired: Black Women's Health Activism in America, 1890–1950*. Philadelphia: University of Pennsylvania Press, 1995.
Smith, Valerie. *Self-Discovery and Authority in Afro-American Narrative*. Cambridge, MA: Harvard University Press, 1987.
Smith-Rosenberg, Carroll. *Disorderly Conduct: Visions of Gender in Victorian America*. Oxford: Oxford University Press, 1986.
Snorton, C. Riley. *Black on Both Sides: A Racial History of Trans Identity*. Minneapolis: University of Minnesota Press, 2017.
Sorisio, Carolyn. *Fleshing Out America: Race, Gender, and the Politics of the Body in American Literature, 1833–1879*. Athens: University of Georgia Press, 2002.
Steele, Jeffrey. "Sentimental Transcendentalism and Political Affect: Child and Fuller in New York." In *Toward a Female Genealogy of Transcendentalism*, edited by Jana L. Argersinger and Phyllis Cole, 207–26. Athens: University of Georgia Press, 2014.
Stoler, Ann Laura. *Race and the Education of Desire: Foucault's History of Sexuality and the Colonial Order of Things*. Durham, NC: Duke University Press, 1995.
Stone, Andrea. *Black Well-Being: Health and Selfhood in Antebellum Black Literature*. Gainesville: University Press of Florida, 2016.
Strings, Sabrina. *Fearing the Black Body: The Racial Origins of Fat Phobia*. New York: New York University Press, 2019.
Sussman, Robert Wald. *The Myth of Race: The Troubling Persistence of an Unscientific Idea*. Cambridge, MA: Harvard University Press, 2014.
Tate, Claudia. *Black Women Writers at Work*. New York: Continuum, 1983.
Taylor, Amy Murrell. *Embattled Freedom: Journeys through the Civil War's Slave Refugee Camps*. Chapel Hill: University of North Carolina Press, 2018.

Teuton, Sean Kicummah. "Disability in Indigenous North America: In Memory of William Sherman Fox." In *The World of Indigenous North America*, edited by Robert Warrior, 569–94. New York: Routledge, 2014.

———. "The Indigenous Body in American Literature." In *The Cambridge Companion to American Literature and the Body*, edited by Travis M. Foster, 210–26. Cambridge: Cambridge University Press, 2022.

Titus, Mary. "'This Poisonous System': Social Ills, Bodily Ills, and Incidents in the Life of a Slave Girl." In *Harriet Jacobs and Incidents in the Life of a Slave Girl: New Critical Essays*, edited by Deborah M. Garfield and Rafia Zafar, 199–215. Cambridge: Cambridge University Press, 1996.

Todd, Jan. *Physical Culture and the Body Beautiful: Purposive Exercise in the Lives of American Women, 1800–1870*. Macon, GA: Mercer University Press, 1998.

Tolentino, Jia. "Always Be Optimizing." In *Trick Mirror: Reflections on Self-Delusion*, 63–94. New York: Random House, 2019.

Tompkins, Kyla Wazana. *Racial Indigestion: Eating Bodies in the 19th Century*. New York: New York University Press, 2012.

Tonkovich, Nicole. *Domesticity with a Difference: The Nonfiction of Catharine Beecher, Sarah J. Hale, Fanny Fern, and Margaret Fuller*. Jackson: University Press of Mississippi, 1997.

Tyler, Dennis. *Disabilities of the Color Line: Redressing Antiblackness from Slavery to the Present*. New York: New York University Press, 2022.

Urban, Andrew. *Brokering Servitude: Migration and the Politics of Domestic Labor during the Long Nineteenth Century*. New York: New York University Press, 2017.

Valenčius, Conevery Bolton. *The Health of the Country: How American Settlers Understood Themselves and Their Land*. New York: Basic Books, 2002.

Verbrugge, Martha H. *Active Bodies: A History of Women's Physical Education in Twentieth-Century America*. New York: Oxford University Press, 2012.

Vertinsky, Patricia Anne. *The Eternally Wounded Woman: Women, Doctors, and Exercise in the Late Nineteenth Century*. Manchester: Manchester University Press, 1990.

Vetter, Lisa Pace. *The Political Thought of America's Founding Feminists*. New York: New York University Press, 2017.

Walker, Alice. *In Search of Our Mothers' Gardens: Womanist Prose*. Boston: Houghton Mifflin Harcourt, 2004.

Wallace-Sanders, Kimberly. *Mammy: A Century of Race, Gender, and Southern Memory*. Ann Arbor: University of Michigan Press, 2008.

Wallach, Glenn. *Obedient Sons: The Discourse of Youth and Generations in American Culture, 1630–1860*. Amherst: University of Massachusetts Press, 1997.

Washington, Harriet A. *Medical Apartheid: The Dark History of Medical Experimentation on Black Americans from Colonial Times to the Present*. New York: Anchor, 2008.

Weiner, Marli F., and Mazie Hough. *Sex, Sickness, and Slavery: Illness in the Antebellum South*. Urbana: University of Illinois Press, 2012.

Wendell, Susan. *The Rejected Body: Feminist Philosophical Reflections on Disability*. London: Routledge, 1996.

Wexler, Laura. *Tender Violence: Domestic Visions in an Age of U.S. Imperialism*. Chapel Hill: University of North Carolina Press, 2000.

Widmer, Edward L. *Young America: The Flowering of Democracy in New York City*. New York: Oxford University Press, 1999.

Wiegman, Robyn. *American Anatomies: Theorizing Race and Gender*. Durham, NC: Duke University Press, 1995.

Woolford, Andrew John. *This Benevolent Experiment: Indigenous Boarding Schools, Genocide, and Redress in Canada and the United States*. Lincoln: University of Nebraska Press, 2015.

Wright, Nazera Sadiq. *Black Girlhood in the Nineteenth Century*. Urbana: University of Illinois Press, 2016.

Yellin, Jean Fagan. *Harriet Jacobs: A Life*. New York: Basic Civitas, 2004.

———, ed. *The Harriet Jacobs Family Papers*. Chapel Hill: University of North Carolina Press, 2008.

Zaborskis, Mary. *Queer Childhoods: Institutional Futures of Indigeneity, Race, and Disability*. New York: New York University Press, 2024.

Journal Articles

Arvin, Maile. "Indigenous Feminist Notes on Embodying Alliance against Settler Colonialism." *Meridians* 18, no. 2 (2019): 335–57.

Baker, Lee D. "The Racist Anti-Racism of American Anthropology." *Transforming Anthropology* 29, no. 2 (2021): 127–42.

Baker, Stephanie Alice. "Alt. Health Influencers: How Wellness Culture and Web Culture Have Been Weaponised to Promote Conspiracy Theories and Far-Right Extremism during the COVID-19 Pandemic." *European Journal of Cultural Studies* 25, no. 1 (2022): 3–24.

Baynton, Douglas. "Slaves, Immigrants, and Suffragists: The Uses of Disability in Citizenship Debates." *PMLA* 120, no. 2 (2005): 562–67.

Bederman, Gail. "Revisiting Nashoba: Slavery, Utopia, and Frances Wright in America, 1818–1826." *American Literary History* 17, no. 3 (2005): 438–59.

Belasco, Susan. "'The Animating Influences of Discord': Margaret Fuller in 1844." *Legacy* 20, nos. 1/2 (2003): 76–93.

Bernardin, Susan. "The Lessons of a Sentimental Education: Zitkala-Ša's Autobiographical Narratives." *Western American Literature* 32, no. 3 (1997): 212–38.

Berry, Sarah L. "'[No] Doctor but My Master': Health Reform and Antislavery Rhetoric in Harriet Jacobs's Incidents in the Life of a Slave Girl." *Journal of Medical Humanities* 35, no. 1 (2014): 1–18.

Branch, Michael P., and Jessica Pierce. "'Another Name for Health': Thoreau and Modern Medicine." *Literature and Medicine* 15, no. 1 (1996): 129–45.

Breau, Elizabeth. "Identifying Satire: Our Nig." *Callaloo* 16, no. 2 (1993): 455–65.

Burt, Ryan. "'Death beneath This Semblance of Civilization': Reading Zitkala-Sa and the Imperial Imagination of the Romantic Revival." *Arizona Quarterly: A Journal of American Literature, Culture, and Theory* 66, no. 2 (2010): 59–88.

Carmody, Todd. "In Spite of Handicaps: The Disability History of Racial Uplift." *American Literary History* 27, no. 1 (2015): 56–78.

Chapman, Chris. "Colonialism, Disability, and Possible Lives: The Residential Treatment of Children Whose Parents Survived Indian Residential Schools." *Journal of Progressive Human Services* 23, no. 2 (2012): 127–58.

Cope, Virginia. "'I Verily Believed Myself to Be a Free Woman': Harriet Jacobs's Journey into Capitalism." *African American Review* 38, no. 1 (2004): 5–20.

Cowing, Jess L. "Occupied Land Is an Access Issue: Interventions in Feminist Disability Studies and Narratives of Indigenous Activism." *Journal of Feminist Scholarship* 17, no. 17 (2020): 9–25.

Cowing, Jess L. Wilcox. "Crip Interventions in Zitkála-Šá's Boarding School Stories." *CUSP: Late Nineteenth and Early Twentieth Century Cultures* 2, no. 2 (2024): 219–29.

Crawford, Robert. "Healthism and the Medicalization of Everyday Life." *International Journal of Health Services* 10, no. 3 (1980): 365–88.

Davis, Cynthia J. "Concerning Children: Charlotte Perkins Gilman, Mothering, and Biography." *Victorian Review* 27, no. 1 (2001): 102–15.

———. "Margaret Fuller, Body and Soul." *American Literature* 71, no. 1 (1999): 31–56.

———. "Speaking the Body's Pain: Harriet Wilson's Our Nig." *African American Review* 27, no. 3 (1993): 391–404.

Diran, Ingrid. "Scenes of Speculation: Harriet Jacobs and the Biopolitics of Human Capital." *American Quarterly* 71, no. 3 (2019): 697–718.

Dudley, Rachel. "Toward an Understanding of the 'Medical Plantation' as a Cultural Location of Disability." *Disability Studies Quarterly* 32, no. 4 (2012).

Dunn, Halbert L. "What High-Level Wellness Means." *Canadian Journal of Public Health/Revue Canadienne de Santé Publique* 50, no. 11 (1959): 447–57.

Edelstein, Sari. "Reading Age beyond Childhood." *ESQ: A Journal of Nineteenth-Century American Literature and Culture* 62, no. 1 (2016): 122–27.

Elman, Julie Passanante. "Slothful Movements: Disability, Acceleration, and Capacity Feminism in Disney's Zootopia (2016)." *Feminist Media Studies*, December 9, 2020, 1–18.

Garland-Thomson, Rosemarie. "Misfits: A Feminist Materialist Disability Concept." *Hypatia* 26, no. 3 (2011): 591–609.

Ginzberg, Lori D. "'The Hearts of Your Readers Will Shudder': Fanny Wright, Infidelity, and American Freethought." *American Quarterly* 46, no. 2 (1994): 195–226.

Gomaa, Sally. "Writing to 'Virtuous' and 'Gentle' Readers: The Problem of Pain in Harriet Jacobs's 'Incidents' and Harriet Wilson's 'Sketches.'" *African American Review* 43, nos. 2/3 (2009): 371–81.

Grimm, Robert Thornton. "Forerunners for a Domestic Revolution: Jane Addams, Charlotte Perkins Gilman, and the Ideology of Childhood, 1900–1916." *Illinois Historical Journal* 90, no. 1 (1997): 47–64.

Henkle, Alex. "'Leaves on the Trees': Ecological Placemaking and Dakota Identity in Zitkala-Ša and Elizabeth Cook-Lynn." *Studies in American Indian Literatures* 35, no. 3 (2023): 124–45.

Herndl, Diane Price. "The Invisible (Invalid) Woman: African-American Women, Illness, and Nineteenth-Century Narrative." *Women's Studies* 24, no. 6 (1995): 553–72.

Hines, Michael. "'They Do Not Know How to Play': Reformers' Expectations and Children's Realities on the First Progressive Playgrounds of Chicago." *Journal of the History of Childhood and Youth* 10, no. 2 (2017): 206–27.

Hovet, Ted. "Harriet Martineau's Exceptional American Narratives: Harriet Beecher Stowe, John Brown, and the 'Redemption of Your National Soul.'" *American Studies* 48, no. 1 (2007): 63–76.

Hudak, Jennifer. "The Social Inventor: Charlotte Perkins Gilman and the (Re)Production of Perfection." *Women's Studies* 32, no. 4 (2003): 455–77.

Hurst, C. Michael. "Bodies in Transition: Transcendental Feminism in Margaret Fuller's Woman in the Nineteenth Century." *Arizona Quarterly: A Journal of American Literature, Culture, and Theory* 66, no. 4 (2010): 1–32.

Kaplan, Amy. "Manifest Domesticity." *American Literature* 70, no. 3 (1998): 581–606.

Kelsey, Penelope. "Disability and Native North American Boarding School Narratives: Madonna Swan and Sioux Sanitorium." *Journal of Literary & Cultural Disability Studies* 7, no. 2 (2013): 195–212.

Kerber, Linda. "The Republican Mother: Women and the Enlightenment—An American Perspective." *American Quarterly* 28, no. 2 (1976): 187–205.

Kim, Jina B., and Sami Schalk. "Reclaiming the Radical Politics of Self-Care: A Crip-of-Color Critique." *South Atlantic Quarterly* 120, no. 2 (2021): 325–42.

Kirkland, Anna. "Critical Perspectives on Wellness." *Journal of Health Politics, Policy and Law* 39, no. 5 (2014): 971–88.

Knight, Denise D. "Charlotte Perkins Gilman and the Shadow of Racism." *American Literary Realism* 32, no. 2 (2000): 159–69.

Kreiger, Georgia. "Playing Dead: Harriet Jacobs's Survival Strategy in 'Incidents in the Life of a Slave Girl.'" *African American Review* 42, nos. 3/4 (2008): 607–21.

Lanser, Susan S. "Feminist Criticism, 'The Yellow Wallpaper,' and the Politics of Color in America." *Feminist Studies* 15, no. 3 (1989): 415–41.

Leveen, Lois. "Dwelling in the House of Oppression: The Spatial, Racial, and Textual Dynamics of Harriet Wilson's Our Nig." *African American Review* 35, no. 4 (2001): 561–80.

Lomawaima, K. Tsianina. "Domesticity in the Federal Indian Schools: The Power of Authority over Mind and Body." *American Ethnologist* 20, no. 2 (1993): 227–40.

———. "Estelle Reel, Superintendent of Indian Schools, 1898–1910: Politics, Curriculum, and Land." *Journal of American Indian Education* 35, no. 3 (1996): 5–31.

Lott, Patricia Ann. "Unweepable Wounds Unwept: Mother Loss, Mourning, and Melancholia in Harriet E. Wilson's Our Nig." *Meridians* 21, no. 2 (2022): 480–505.

Lovell, Thomas B. "By Dint of Labor and Economy: Harriet Jacobs, Harriet Wilson, and the Salutary View of Wage Labor." *Arizona Quarterly: A Journal of American Literature, Culture, and Theory* 52, no. 2 (1996): 1–32.

MacBain, Tiffany Aldrich. "Cont(r)Acting Whiteness: The Language of Contagion in the Autobiographical Essays of Zitkala-Ša." *Arizona Quarterly: A Journal of American Literature, Culture, and Theory* 68, no. 3 (2012): 55–69.

May, Vivian, and Beth Ferri. "Fixated on Ability: Questioning Ableist Metaphors in Feminist Theories of Resistance." *Prose Studies* 27 (2005): 120–40.

McCrary, Lorraine Krall. "From Hull-House to Herland: Engaged and Extended Care in Jane Addams and Charlotte Perkins Gilman." *Politics & Gender* 15, no. 1 (2019): 62–82.

McIntyre, Adrianna, Nicholas Bagley, Austin Frakt, and Aaron Carroll. "The Dubious Empirical and Legal Foundations of Wellness Programs." *Health Matrix: The Journal of Law-Medicine* 27, no. 1 (2017): 59.

Mickey, Ethel L. "'"Eat, Pray, Love" Bullshit': Women's Empowerment through Wellness at an Elite Professional Conference." *Journal of Contemporary Ethnography* 48, no. 1 (2019): 103–27.

Mills, Bruce. "Lydia Maria Child and the Endings to Harriet Jacobs's Incidents in the Life of a Slave Girl." *American Literature* 64, no. 2 (1992): 255–72.

Morantz, Regina Markell. "Making Women Modern: Middle-Class Women and Health Reform in 19th Century America." *Journal of Social History* 10, no. 4 (1977): 490–507.

Morgensen, Scott Lauria. "The Biopolitics of Settler Colonialism: Right Here, Right Now." *Settler Colonial Studies* 1, no. 1 (2011): 52–76.

Murison, Justine S. "The Tyranny of Sleep: Somnambulism, Moral Citizenship, and Charles Brockden Brown's 'Edgar Huntly.'" *Early American Literature* 44, no. 2 (2009): 243–70.

Murphy, Maureen. "The Irish Servant Girl in Literature." *Writing Ulster* 5 (1998): 133–47.

O'Neill, Rachel. "Pursuing 'Wellness': Considerations for Media Studies." *Television & New Media* 21, no. 6 (2020): 628–34.

Ousley, Laurie. "The Business of Housekeeping: The Mistress, the Domestic Worker, and the Construction of Class." *Legacy* 23, no. 2 (2006): 132–47.

Palumbo-DeSimone, Christine. "'Kitchen Queens' and 'Tributary Housekeepers': Irish Servant Stories in Nineteenth-Century Women's Magazine Fiction." *Tulsa Studies in Women's Literature* 33, no. 2 (2014): 77–101.

Park, Roberta J. "The Attitudes of Leading New England Transcendentalists toward Healthful Exercise, Active Recreations and Proper Care of the Body: 1830–1860." *Journal of Sport History* 4, no. 1 (1977): 34–50.

———. "'Embodied Selves': The Rise and Development of Concern for Physical Education, Active Games and Recreation for American Women, 1776–1865." *International Journal of the History of Sport* 24, no. 12 (2007): 1508–42.

Piep, Karsten H. "'Nothing New under the Sun': Postsentimental Conflict in Harriet E. Wilson's Our Nig." *Colloquy* 11 (2006): 178–94.

Pitts, Yvonne. "Disability, Scientific Authority, and Women's Political Participation at the Turn of the Twentieth-Century United States." *Journal of Women's History* 24, no. 2 (2012): 37–61.

Plasencia, Sam. "Staging Enfleshment: Toward Lines of Flight in Harriet Wilson's Our Nig; or, Sketches from the Life of a Free Black." *Legacy: A Journal of American Women Writers* 37, no. 2 (2020): 189–212.

Redmond, C. Daniel. "The Sartorial Indian: Zitkala-Ša, Clothing, and Resistance to Colonization." *Studies in American Indian Literatures* 28, no. 3 (2016): 52–80.

Reiss, Benjamin. "Sleeping at Walden Pond: Thoreau, Abnormal Temporality, and the Modern Body." *American Literature* 85, no. 1 (2013): 5–31.

Rifkin, Mark. "Indigenizing Agamben: Rethinking Sovereignty in Light of the 'Peculiar' Status of Native Peoples." *Cultural Critique* 73, no. 1 (2009): 88-124.

Robbins, Sarah. "Periodizing Authorship, Characterizing Genre: Catharine Maria Sedgwick's Benevolent Literacy Narratives." *American Literature* 76, no. 1 (2004): 1-29.

Schalk, Sami. "Metaphorically Speaking: Ableist Metaphors in Feminist Writing." *Disability Studies Quarterly* 33, no. 4 (2013).

Schalk, Sami, and Jina B. Kim. "Integrating Race, Transforming Feminist Disability Studies." *Signs: Journal of Women in Culture and Society* 46, no. 1 (2020): 31-55.

Schneiderhan, Erik. "Pragmatism and Empirical Sociology: The Case of Jane Addams and Hull-House, 1889-1895." *Theory and Society* 40, no. 6 (2011): 589-617.

Scholl, Lesa. "Mediation and Expansion: Harriet Martineau's Travels in America." *Women's History Review* 18, no. 5 (2009): 819-33.

Seigfried, Charlene Haddock. "Socializing Democracy: Jane Addams and John Dewey." *Philosophy of the Social Sciences* 29, no. 2 (1999): 207-30.

Senier, Siobhan. "Disability, Blackness, and Indigeneity: An Invitation to a Conversation." *CLA Journal* 64, no. 1 (2021): 166-73.

Short, Gretchen. "Harriet Wilson's *Our Nig* and the Labor of Citizenship." *Arizona Quarterly: A Journal of American Literature, Culture, and Theory* 57, no. 3 (2001): 1-27.

Spack, Ruth. "Dis/Engagement: Zitkala-Ša's Letters to Carlos Montezuma, 1901-1902." *MELUS* 26, no. 1 (2001): 173-204.

———. "Re-Visioning Sioux Women: Zitkala-Ša's Revolutionary American Indian Stories." *Legacy* 14, no. 1 (1997): 25-42.

Spillers, Hortense J. "Mama's Baby, Papa's Maybe: An American Grammar Book." *Diacritics* 17, no. 2 (1987): 65-81.

Stern, Julia. "Excavating Genre in *Our Nig*." *American Literature* 67, no. 3 (1995): 439-66.

Suhr-Sytsma, Mandy. "Spirits from Another Realm, Activists in Their Own Right: The Figure of the Yankton/Romantic Child in Zitkala-Sa's Work." *Children's Literature* 42, no. 1 (2014): 136-68.

Tan, Annabel X., Jessica A. Hinman, Hoda S. Abdel Magid, Lorene M. Nelson, and Michelle C. Odden. "Association between Income Inequality and County-Level COVID-19 Cases and Deaths in the US." *JAMA Network Open* 4, no. 5 (2021): e218799.

Tavera, Stephanie Peebles. "Her Body, Herland: Reproductive Health and Dis/Topian Satire in Charlotte Perkins Gilman." *Utopian Studies* 29, no. 1 (2018): 1-20.

Till, Christopher. "Creating 'Automatic Subjects': Corporate Wellness and Self-Tracking." *Health* 23, no. 4 (2019): 418-35.

Trennert, Robert A. "Educating Indian Girls at Nonreservation Boarding Schools, 1878-1920." *Western Historical Quarterly* 13, no. 3 (1982): 271-90.

———. "Selling Indian Education at World's Fairs and Expositions, 1893-1904." *American Indian Quarterly* 11, no. 3 (1987): 203-20.

Walter, Krista. "Surviving in the Garret: Harriet Jacobs and the Critique of Sentiment." *ATQ* 8, no. 3 (1994): 189-210.

Walters, Shannon. "Crip Mammy: Complicating Race, Gender, and Care in *The Ride Together*." *Journal of Literary & Cultural Disability Studies* 11, no. 4 (2017): 477-93.

Weinbaum, Alys Eve. "Writing Feminist Genealogy: Charlotte Perkins Gilman, Racial Nationalism, and the Reproduction of Maternalist Feminism." *Feminist Studies* 27, no. 2 (2001): 271–302.

White, Barbara A. "'Our Nig' and the She-Devil: New Information about Harriet Wilson and the 'Bellmont' Family." *American Literature* 65, no. 1 (1993): 19–52.

Zink, Amanda J. "Carlisle's Writing Circle: Boarding School Texts and the Decolonization of Domesticity." *Studies in American Indian Literatures* 27, no. 4 (2015): 37–65.

Index

Abate, Michelle Ann, 116, 164n157
ableism, 32–33, 67–68
abolition movement, 26–27, 58–60, 139n15, 152n124. *See also* enslaved persons; slavery
Addams, Jane, 12, 13, 101–3, 107–13, 122, 126
Advice to Young Mothers on the Physical Education of Children (Moore), 4
Alaimo, Stacey, 35
Alcott, Amos Bronson, 28
Alcott, Louisa May, 5, 28
alternative embodiments, 96–99
American apathy, 21–27
American Association for the Advancement of Physical Education, 100
American Journal of Sociology, 124
apathy, 21–27
An Appeal in Favor of That Class of Americans Called Africans (Child), 67
assimilationist education, 154n11. *See also* Native people
asylum, 95–96. *See also* incarceration
"Autobiographical Romance" (Fuller), 29
Autobiography (Martineau), 26–27
Ayurvedic diet, 132–33

Bacon, Amanda Chantal, 128–29
Bancroft, Jessie Hubbell, 100–101
Barbie Wellness Collection, 127
Baynton, Douglas, 104
Bederman, Gail, 16
Beecher, Catharine, 4–5, 11, 27, 39–43, 59, 90
Ben-Moshe, Liat, 81, 95
"biological engineering," 2, 103–8
Black communities: Jacobs' work for, 11–12, 70–79; legacy of exhaustion in, 135; physical education in, 6, 7; presumed fitness of women in, 2; Stanley's work on wellness in, 131, 134, 135; Walker on womanism in, 168n57; Wilson's *Our Nig* on, 49–57, 146nn84–86, 147n97, 147n100, 147nn92–93. *See also* racial capitalism; racial science
Blackwell, Elizabeth, 1
Blaikie, William, 107, 117
Blumenthal, Rachel A., 30
Boas, Franz, 105
Bonnin, Gertrude. *See* Zitkala-Ša
Boster, Dea H., 66
Boston Normal School of Gymnastics (BNSG), 6
Boston Women's Health Collective, 130
Boyd, Neva, 109, 114
Brodesser-Akner, Taffy, 130
Burbick, Joan, 8
Burch, Susan, 33, 83
Bureau of Immigration, 104
Bureau of Indian Affairs, 80
Burgess, Marianna, 12, 86
Byrd, Jodi, 154n3

Canton Asylum, 95–96
capacity feminism, 9–10
capitalism, 129–31, 134–35, 144nn33–34
Carby, Hazel, 62
caregiving, 60–64, 70–79
Carlisle Indian Industrial School, 12, 80–99, 155n26, 156n43
Carmody, Todd, 78
Cartwright, Samuel, 60
Channing, William Ellery, 145n35
Charities and the Commons (Addams), 115

189

Chautauqua Normal School of Physical Education, 83
Chicago Relief and Aid Society, 161n62
Chicago School for Playground Workers, 109, 161n65
Child, Lydia Maria, 4, 58, 63, 67, 139n15, 149n11
childcare programs, 108–9, 161n62
child-culture, 116–26, 164n178
Chinese Exclusion Act (1882), 159n22
Choate, John Nicholas, 83
chronic illness, 131–32, 135, 167n28. *See also* illness
citizenship, 100–126
class mobility, 43–49, 144nn33–34
clothing, 91–92
Coffin, Joshua, 67
Cogan, Frances, 64
Collective Napping Experience, 135
colonial violence, 80. *See also* Black communities; capitalism; Carlisle Indian Industrial School; Native people; slavery
"Colored Refugees in Our Camps" (Jacobs), 75
Concerning Children (Gilman), 118–19
contraband camps, 58–59, 70–79. *See also* enslaved persons
Cooper, James Fenimore, 16
Cope, Virginia, 68
cosmopolitanism, 108–16
A Course of Calisthenics for Young Ladies (anonymous), 4, 5
Course of Study for the Indian Schools of the United States (Reel), 87, 158n100
COVID-19 pandemic, 128–29
Cowing, Jess L. Wilcox, 33, 81, 94
Crampton, Charles Ward, 106–7
Crawford, Robert, 128
criminality, 165n203, 165n205
The Crux (Gilman), 118
Cullen, William, 17
cure rhetoric, 78–79

Davenport, Charles, 104
Davis, Cynthia J., 30, 146n85
debility (term), 154n12
Democracy and Social Ethics (Addams), 110
Democracy in America (Tocqueville), 22
Department of Indian Education (NEA), 89
Dewey, John, 109
Dewey, Mary, 43–49
disability pedagogies, 2, 9, 10, 12, 32, 66, 78, 82, 93, 97–99, 160n54. *See also* ableism; illness
divine instinct of maternity, 117
domesticity, 38–39, 137n9
Domestic Manners of the Americans (Trollope), 22
domestic manuals, 4, 37–43, 127–28, 134
domestic novels, 43–57
domestic workers, 39–43, 62, 144n23
Donokor, Crystal S., 72
Doty, Josh, 10
Douglass, Frederick, 58, 59, 74
Dow, Marietta, 162n117
DreamSpace, 135, 168n58
Dudden, Faye, 41
Duffin, James W., 150n53
Dunn, Halbert L., 128
Duyckinck, Evert, 15

economic paternalism, 144n33. *See also* capitalism
Edelstein, Sari, 14–15
Ellis Island, 103–4
Elman, Julia Passanante, 9
embodiments, 8–9, 96–99. *See also* disability pedagogies; illness; physical education
Emerson, Ralph Waldo, 33
Émile; or, On Education (Rousseau), 29
empowerment, 9–10, 129
enslaved persons, 42, 58–79. *See also* abolition movement; contraband camps; slavery
Erevelles, Nirmala, 73

An Essay on the Principle of Population (Malthus), 21
essentialism, 1, 2, 6, 7, 32–33, 35, 45, 54, 59, 61, 114
eugenics, 8, 103–6, 116–26, 163n124
Every Body Yoga (Stanley), 134
exercise. *See* physical education

The Family Nurse (Child), 72
Farmer's Cabinet (newspaper), 147n92
Farrar, Eliza Ware, 37–39
female frailty, 1, 2, 19, 24, 25, 33, 66, 94, 130
Fish, Cheryl J., 31–32
fitness (term), 9
Forbes (magazine), 129
"A Fourteen Year Old Girl's Good Advice" (Burgess), 86–87
frailty, 1, 2, 19, 24, 25, 33, 66, 94, 130
The Freedmen's Book (Child), 71
Freedmen's Record (journal), 77, 78, 153n144
fugitive science, 3
Fuller, Margaret, 3, 11, 15, 16, 26–36, 81, 126

Galton, Francis, 107
"A Garden of Babies" (Gilman), 118, 119
Garland-Thomson, Rosemarie, 9
geography of health (concept), 31
Gilman, Charlotte Perkins, 13, 101, 116–26, 159n14; autobiography of, 116; on child-culture, 116, 118–19, 164n178; on female frailty, 130; *Herland*, 102, 120, 121, 124, 125, 164n154, 164n157; "Immigration, Importation, and Our Fathers," 126; as mother, 163n129; *Moving the Mountain*, 119, 120, 124; on national physical education, 108; "A Suggestion on the Negro Problem," 125–26; *What Our Girls Ought to Know*, 117; *With Her in Ourland*, 122–23; *Women and Economics*, 117–18; *The Yellow Wall Paper*, 164n178
"Girls Read This" (Burgess), 86

Glenn, Evelyn Nagano, 38
Gliddon, George R., 61
Goodlad, Lauren M. E., 26
Goop, 128, 130
The Gospel of Wellness (Raphael), 130
Graham, Sylvester, 5
Grigg, Amanda J., 130
Grimké, Angelina Weld, 6
grind culture, 135, 136
Gyles, Rose, 107–8, 109, 114
gymnastics, 5, 6, 163n138. *See also* physical education

Hailmann, William Nicholas, 83
Hall, Prescot F., 105
Hampton Agricultural and Industrial School, 6, 89, 155n27
Harper, Frances Ellen Watkins, 77, 153n137
Harper, Lila Marz, 15
Hartford Female Seminary, 39–40
Hartman, Saidiya V., 66
Harvard University Summer School of Physical Training, 6
Hawthorne, Nathaniel, 15
health: disparities in, 2–3; politics of, 8–10; radical, 3, 13, 130–31, 134–36; Stone on rhetoric of, 149n8; women writing on, 10–13; Wright and Republicanism on, 16–21. *See also* illness; physical education; wellness culture
healthism, 128
health knowledge, 1, 43–49. *See also* health
Heredity in Relation to Eugenics (Davenport), 104
Herland (Gilman), 102, 120, 121, 124, 125, 164n154, 164n157
Herndl, Diane Price, 64
Hersey, Tricia, 131, 135–36, 168n57, 168n58
Higginson, Thomas Wentworth, 143n1
hiking, 32
The History of the Condition of Women (Child), 62

Index 191

Hovet, Ted, 22
"How and Why Women Can and Should Prioritize Their Wellness" (Sinha), 129–30
How to Get Strong and How to Stay So (Blaikie), 107, 117
How to Observe (Martineau), 24
Huber, Sonya, 131–32
Hudak, Jennifer, 126
Hull-House settlement, 12–13, 107–16, 119, 160n57, 162n117
Humaniculture, 119–20
Hunt, Harriot Kezia, 1
Hurst, C. Michael, 27–28

illness, 128–29, 131–32, 135, 167n28. *See also* ableism
Illustrations of Political Economy (Martineau), 21
immigrants and physical education, 101–26
"Immigration, Importation, and Our Fathers" (Gilman), 126
Immigration Act (1917), 159n22
Immigration Commission, 105, 112
Immigration Restriction League, 104
"Impressions of an Indian Childhood" (Zitkala-Ša), 92, 96
incarceration, 74, 82, 85, 95–96, 125, 165n203, 165n205
Incidents in the Life of a Slave Girl (Jacobs), 11, 58–60, 62, 64–70, 75, 149n13
indentured servitude, 49–57
Indian Helper (newspaper), 80, 85, 86, 90
Indigenous womanhood, 33–36, 90–99
Iola Leroy (Harper), 77

Jackson, Shannon, 110
Jacobs, Harriet, 11–12, 58–60, 64–79
Jacobs, Louisa, 11, 77–78, 153n135
Jacobs School, 77

Kafer, Alison, 32
Kaplan, Amy, 5, 38, 144n24
Katanski, Amelia V., 86

Kerber, Linda, 5, 20
Kim, Jina B., 9, 131
Kirkland, Anna, 129, 130
Kolodny, Anette, 34
Kowacura, Stiya, 86

Ladies' Home Journal, 113
Larocca, Amy, 129
Lectures to Women on Anatomy and Physiology (Nichols), 5
Letters from New York (Child), 139n15
Letters to Persons Who Are Engaged in Domestic Service (Beecher), 40, 41
Liberator (newspaper), 61, 71
"Life among the Contrabands" (Jacobs), 71–73
Litchfield Female Academy, 4–5
Little Men (Alcott), 6
Little Women (Alcott), 5
Live and Let Live (Sedgwick), 43–49, 51, 57, 144nn33–35
The Living of Charlotte Perkins Gilman (Gilman), 116
Locke, John, 17, 28–29
Lomawaima, K. Tsianina, 81
Long, Margaret Geneva, 71
Lorde, Audre, 13, 131

Malthus, Robert, 21
Manson, Deborah, 30
Martineau, Harriet, 10, 11, 15, 21–27, 31, 130
Matthews, Cornelius, 15
McCrary, Lorraine Krall, 120
Means and Ends (Sedgwick), 5, 141n106
Metzl, Jonathan, 8
Millar, John, 17
Millar, Robina Craig, 17
Minich, Julie Avril, 3
Minnie's Sacrifice (Harper), 153n137
Monthly Repository (periodical), 22
Moore, Margaret King, 4
moral health, 25
Morton, Samuel, 61
motherhood, 5, 20, 117–19, 163n129

The Mother's Book (Child), 4, 63, 64
Moving the Mountain (Gilman), 119, 120, 124
Mylne, James, 17

Nadler, Stephen, 78
National Anti-Slavery Standard (newspaper), 58, 60, 139n15, 149n19
National Black Women's Health Project, 130
National Education Association (NEA), 89
National Home for the Relief of Destitute Colored Women and Children, 153n135
Native people: assimilationist education for, 154n11; Carlisle Indian Industrial School for, 12, 80–99, 155n26, 156n43; womanhood of, 33–36, 90–99. *See also* Zitkala-Ša
nature, 32–35
New Harmony community, 20–21
A New Home (Kirkland), 139n15
New York Tribune (newspaper) 60
Nichols, Mary Gove, 5
Normal Institute for Physical Training, 5, 6
Normal School of Physical Training, 6
North Star (newspaper), 58, 59, 65, 74
Nott, Josiah Clark, 61

"The Objective Value of a Social Settlement" (Addams), 108
Observations Concerning the Distinction of Ranks in Society (Millar), 17
"Of the Rank and Condition of Women in Different Ages" (Millar), 17
O'Neill, Rachel, 131
"On Female Education" (Martineau), 22–23
On the Mode of Education Proper in a Republic (Rush), 19
O'Sullivan, John, 15
Our Nig (Wilson), 49–57, 146nn84–86, 147n97, 147n100, 147nn92–93

outing system, 89
Owen, Robert, 20

Pain Woman Takes Your Keys (Huber), 131
Paltrow, Gwyneth, 128
Parks, Roberta, 6–7
paternalism, 144n33
The Pedagogy of Physical Training (Crampton), 106
Pestalozzi, Johann Heinrich, 109
Phelps, Almira Hart Lincoln, 2
physical culture movement, 137n10
physical education: Farrar on, 37–39; Fuller on, 26–36; in Hull-House settlement, 12–13, 107–16; of immigrants, 101–26; in Indian boarding schools, 12, 81–99; Phelps on, 2; politics of, 2–8; racial differences in, 6; sex differences in, 73, 83, 86. *See also* embodiments; gymnastics; self-cultivation
Physical Education (Galton), 107
Physical Education and the Preservation of Health (Warren), 30
Pierce, Sarah, 4
Plain Talk and Friendly Advice to Domestics (anonymous), 147n93
A Plan for Improving Female Education (Willard), 14
Posse, Baron, 100
pragmatism, 161n66
Pratt, Richard Henry, 80, 83–84, 94, 98–99
"Prize Children" (Gilman), 116
Puar, Jasbir, 9, 154n12
"The Public School and the Immigrant Child" (Addams), 114–15
Purkiss, Ava, 7

queerness, 164n154. *See also* sexuality

racial capitalism, 135. *See also* slavery
racial science, 60–64
radical health, 3, 13, 130–31, 134–36

Index 193

Raphael, Rina, 130
Recreation Training School, 109
Red Man and Helper (newspaper), 95
Red Man and Helper (Zitkala-Ša), 98
Redmond, C. Daniel, 92
Reel, Estelle, 12, 87, 92, 156n40
reform physiology, 5
rehabilitation, 78
repatriation, 135
"Report on the Diseases and Physical Peculiarities of the Negro Race" (Cartwright), 60
republicanism, 16–21
republican motherhood, 5, 20
rest, 135, 165n207
Rest Is Resistance (Hersey), 135
Retrospect of Western Travel (Martineau), 21
Richards, Josephine E., 89
rivers, 96, 158n104
Rochester Anti-Slavery Reading Room, 62
Róisín, Fariha, 131, 132, 133, 134
Roosevelt, Theodore, 85–86
Rose, Ernestine, 1–2
Rosowski, Susan J., 30
Rousseau, Jean-Jacques, 29
Rusert, Britt, 3, 60
Rush, Benjamin, 17, 19

Sanger, Margaret, 8, 103
Sargent, Dudley Allen, 6, 101, 106–7, 160n50, 160n54, 165n205
Sargent, F. P., 104
Sargent School of Physical Education, 6, 107, 109
Schalk, Sami, 9, 131
"The School Days of an Indian Girl" (Zitkala-Ša), 90–91
School Gymnastics (Bancroft), 100
Schuller, Kyla, 8, 30, 81
scientific racism, 60–64
Sedgwick, Catharine Maria, 4, 5, 27, 39, 43–49
self-acceptance, 133–34

self-care, 13, 64–70, 127, 130–31, 167n30. *See also* wellness culture
self-cultivation, 3–6, 9, 27–28, 35. *See also* physical education
settlement movement, 160n57. *See also* Hull-House settlement
settler colonialism and education, 11, 16, 31, 33, 81–83, 97, 157n84. *See also* Carlisle Indian Industrial School; Native people
settler feminism, 87, 157n84
sexism, 3, 29–30, 34
sexuality, 7, 104, 115, 146n85, 164n154
sexual violence, 7, 63, 124
Shape (magazine), 132–33
Short, Gretchen, 50
Sigourney, Lydia, 4
Simmons, Gertrude. *See* Zitkala-Ša
slavery, 26, 58–59, 60–64. *See also* abolition movement; enslaved persons; racial capitalism
Slavery Illustrated in Its Effects upon Women and Domestic Society (Bourne), 62
Smith, Charles Hamilton, 54, 61
Smith, Valerie, 64
Snorton, C. Riley, 79
Society in America (Martineau), 16, 21, 31
Society of Friends, 70
Some Thoughts Concerning Education (Locke), 17, 28–29
Sorisio, Carolyn, 30
The Spirit of Youth and the City Streets (Addams), 113, 162n97
Stanley, Jessamyn, 131, 133–34, 135
Starr, Ellen Gates, 108
Steinem, Gloria, 138n34
Stevenson, Hannah, 153n133
Stewart, Maria W., 74
Stiya (Burgess), 86
Stoler, Ann Laura, 154n4
Stowe, Harriet Beecher, 39

Studio Ānanda, 133
Studley, Mary J., 117
suffrage, 8, 10
"A Suggestion on the Negro Problem" (Gilman), 125–26
Summer on the Lakes (Fuller), 11, 16, 27–36
The Sun Dance Opera (Zitkala-Ša), 95
survival, 64–70
Sweden, 100, 163n138

Talbot, Eugene, 104–5
Temple School, 28
Teuton, Sean Kicummah, 34, 83
Thompson, William Grant, 83, 155nn26–27
Thoreau, Henry David, 28, 31
Titus, Mary, 65
Tocqueville, Alexis de, 22
Todd, Jan, 7
Tolentino, Jia, 128
Tompkins, Kyla Wazana, 3–4, 146n84
transcendentalism, 11, 26, 27, 28, 30, 33, 142nn107–8
Travels in Canada, and the United States, in 1816 and 1817 (Hall), 18
A Treatise on Domestic Economy (Beecher), 40, 41–42
Trollope, Frances, 22
Troy Female Seminary, 139n1
Tuskegee Institute, 6
Twenty Years at Hull-House (Addams), 110–11, 112, 114
Types of Mankind (Nott and Gliddon), 61

Uncle Tom's Cabin (Stowe), 39
"The Underbelly" project, 133
universal education, 19–20

Valenčius, Conevery Bolton, 31
Verbrugge, Martha, 7, 106
Vertinsky, Patricia, 7
Vetter, Lisa Pace, 19

Views of Society and Manners in America (Wright), 16–21
A Vindication on the Rights of Woman (Wollstonecraft), 19
voting rights, 8, 10

Walden (Thoreau), 32
Walker, Alice, 168n57
Ward, Robert DeCourcey, 104
Warren, John C., 30
"A Warrior's Daughter" (Zitkala-Ša), 158n100
wellness culture, 13, 127–34, 136
Wendell, Susan, 9
"What High-Level Wellness Means" (Dunn), 128
What Our Girls Ought to Know (Studley), 117
white nationalism, 3, 7
White's Manual Labor Institute, 90, 91
white supremacy, 122, 134, 135. *See also* racial capitalism
white womanhood: embodied norms of, 32, 144n12; future of, 14–16; presumed frailty of, 2, 33; suffragists and exclusion by, 8
Whitman, Walt, 15
Who Is Wellness For? (Róisín), 132
"Why I Am a Pagan" (Zitkala-Ša), 96–98, 158n104
Willard, Emma, 14, 139n1
Wilson, Harriet, 39, 49–57, 147n92, 147nn92–93
With Her in Ourland (Gilman), 122–23
Wollstonecraft, Mary, 19
Woman in the Nineteenth Century (Fuller), 27–28
womanism, 168n57
Woman's Rights Convention (1852), 1
Women and Economics (Gilman), 117–18
women's health. *See* health
Women's Medical College, 1

Woodhull, Victoria, 8, 103
Wright, Frances, 10, 15, 16–21, 31
writing health, 10–13

The Yellow Wall Paper (Gilman), 164n178, 165n207
YMCA (Young Men's Christian Association), 85
yoga, 127, 131–34

Yoke (Stanley), 134
The Young Lady's Friend (Farrar), 37
"Your Complete Guide to the Ayurvedic Diet" (Falk), 132–33

Zaborski, Mary, 87
Zitkala-Ša, 3, 12, 90–99, 154n6, 154n17, 155n18, 155n21, 157n65, 157n84, 157n87, 158n100

www.ingramcontent.com/pod-product-compliance
Lightning Source LLC
Chambersburg PA
CBHW032214230426
43672CB00011B/2556